HERBAL LORE

K.J. SIMMILL

Contents

Titles by K.J. Simmill

Fiction:

The Forgotten Legacies Series:

Darrienia

The Severaine

Remedy

The Dreamwalker

Non-Fiction:

Herbal Lore

Methods of Extraction
and Application

Extraction

Extraction is the process of obtaining a herbal extract from selected parts of a herb. This can then be added to different things to make anything you need, from candles and incense, to rubs and lotions.

It is better to use fresh herbs for extraction, however, dried herbs can be used but often require additional fluid to be added.

If you are using a number of herbs for a single purpose you can combine them prior to extraction. The general ratio for herb to liquid is 1oz to ¼ pint, the volume of liquid may need to be increased slightly if you are using dried herbs.

If you don't wish to make your own extract, most Apothecary shops and herbalist carry, or can order, extracts and tinctures.

Extracts and tinctures do not have to be added to anything, they can be taken neat if desired, or added to water as a drink.

Application

Application is the method chosen to use your herbal extract, this can be anything from compresses and teas, to candles and incense

Methods of Extraction

Decoction

Information: Used to create an extract from hard parts of a herb such as bark or roots. There are a few exceptions, such as red clover, where this method is more suited. There are also some herbs that work better for a specific purpose when used as a decoction (E.G Country Mallow, Flaxseed, Hyssop etc). Decoctions can be drunk or used to apply the mixture externally by compress or wash, they are also useful for adding to the bath.

Shelf life: Short - Up to 3 days if kept refrigerated. Better for immediate use.

Preparation time: 15 minutes.

Method:

1. Use one pint of water to 1oz of the herb.
2. Cut or crush the herb.
3. Add water to a saucepan.

4. Put on a medium heat and simmer until water has reduced by a quarter to half the initial volume.
5. Place a muslin cloth into a fine mesh sieve and slowly pour the contents of the jar into the sieve to drain into a glass jar.
6. Fold the cloth around the herbs and squeeze any remaining liquid out into the jar.
7. Either use or leave to cool.
8. Once cooled seal and label jar and place in the fridge.

Extract

Information: This can be used on most herbs and is an easy way to create a long-life extract without the use of alcohol. The liquid used to make an extract can be cider vinegar, rice wine vinegar, or vegetable glycerine. Use the ratio 1oz herb to ¼ pint of fluid.

If you wish to use alcohol, then you need to follow the instructions for a tincture.

Shelf life: 3 - 5 years

Preparation time: 4 - 6 weeks

Method:

1. Weigh the jar.
2. Chop the herb finely and add to a sealable glass jar.
3. Weigh the jar again and subtract the initial weight to obtain the weight of the herbs. and calculate the volume of fluid needed. (¼ pint per 1oz herb).
4. Pour the liquid over the herbs.
5. Stir the contents gently to remove any air bubbles.
6. If you are using vinegar it tends to rust metal jar lids

so be sure to place some cling film or baking paper over the jar before placing the lid on.

7. Seal the jar, shake the contents, and remember to add a label so you know what is in there.

8. Place in a dark area, returning every few days to give the mixture a shake - note: if you have used dried herbs you may wish to add a little more fluid after three days as dried herbs take in more moisture.

9. Leave for 4 - 6 weeks.

10. Place a muslin cloth into a fine mesh and slowly pour the contents of the jar into the sieve to drain into a glass bowl.

11. Fold the cloth around the herbs and squeeze any remaining liquid out through the sieve and into the bowl.

12. Funnel the liquid into smaller glass bottles. Be sure to use dark or amber glass to protect the mixture from light and ensure it lasts longer.

13. Label with contents and date, and store in a cool dark place.

Infusion

Information: This can be used for most herbs and is a simple way to make a herbal water which can be drank or applied externally as a wash or compress. Infusions are also useful for adding to a bath. Use the ratio 1oz herb to ¼ pint water. These are best prepared at night to be ready for the next morning.

Shelf life: Short - Up to 3 days if kept refrigerated. Better for immediate use.

Preparation time: 12 hours.

Method:

1. Weigh the jar.
2. Chop the herb and add to a sealable glass jar.
3. Weigh the jar again and subtract the initial weight to obtain the weight of the herbs. and calculate the volume of water needed. (¼ pint per 1oz herb).
4. Add the water to the jar.
5. Seal the jar and place in a cool dark place over night.
6. Place a piece of muslin cloth into a fine mesh sieve and slowly pour the contents of the jar into the sieve to drain into a glass bowl or jar.
7. Fold the cloth around the herbs and squeeze any remaining liquid out through the sieve and into the bowl or jar.
8. Use immediately or place in the fridge.

Tea (Hot infusion)

Information: A tea is one of the more well-known methods of consuming herbs. It is a simple and quick process which draws out the oils and vitamins from a herb. It is best used on softer or finely chopped dried herbs. For bark and roots a decoction is the better method.

Shelf life: 12 hours, but it is better drunk fresh and warm.

Preparation time: 15 minutes.

Method:

1. Add selected herbs into an infuser or sieve and place into a cup.
2. Pour boiling water over the infuser or sieve to fill the cup.
3. Cover the cup and leave for 15 minutes.
4. Place a piece of muslin cloth over a fine mesh sieve

and transfer contents through sieve to another cup to remove any bits.

Note: Some Apothecary shops and herbalists sell empty teabags which can be filled with herbs of your choice. An infuser is a good alternative to these as they are more cost effective and can be reused.

Tincture

Information: This can be used on most herbs and is an easy way to create a long-life extract. This is made using a strong alcohol (80 proof/40%), anything with a strong proof will work, but vodka is the most commonly used alcohol due to its tasteless nature not adding additional flavour to the extract. Use the ratio 1oz herb to ¼ pint alcohol.

If you don't wish to use alcohol, then you need to follow the instructions for an extract.

Shelf life: Long - Several years.

Preparation time: 4 - 6 weeks.

Method:

1. Weigh the jar.
2. Chop the herb finely and add to a sealable glass jar.
3. Weigh the jar again and subtract the initial weight to obtain the weight of the herbs. and calculate the volume of alcohol needed. (¼ pint per 1oz herb).
4. Pour the alcohol over the herbs.
5. Stir the contents gently to remove any air bubbles.
6. Seal the jar, shake the contents, and remember to add a label so you know what is in there.
7. Place in a dark area returning every few days to give the mixture a shake - note: if you have used dried

herbs you may need to add a little more alcohol after
three days as dried herbs take in more moisture.

8. Leave for 4 - 6 weeks.
9. Place a cloth into a fine mesh sieve and slowly pour
   the contents of the jar into the sieve to drain into a
   glass bowl.
10. Fold the cloth around the herbs and squeeze any
   remaining liquid out through the sieve and into the
   bowl.
11. Funnel the liquid into smaller glass bottles. Be sure to
   use dark or amber glass to protect the mixture from
   light and ensure it lasts longer.
12. Label with contents and date, and store in a cool dark
   place.

Methods of Application

Making a Compress

Uses:

Use a hot compress to treat boils, menstrual cramps, muscle pain, rheumatic pain and toothache.

Use a cold compress to treat bruises, fevers, headaches, inflammation and swelling.

Method:

1. Take a bowl of water, for a hot compress use hot water, for cold use refrigerated or iced water.
2. Add 3 - 6 drops of your herbal extract or tincture to the water.
3. Skim your bandage or flannel across the top of the water and wring it out.
4. Apply directly to the area until it has cooled, or warmed, to body temperature, then repeat.

Alternatively, instead of water and an extract you can use a decoction or an infusion without the need to add additional oils and simply warm or cool as required.

Making a Poultice

Uses:

Use a poultice on abscesses, acne, arthritis, bruises, external skin conditions, inflammation, sprains, to draw out foreign objects, and on wounds.

Method:

1. Chop the selected herbs.
2. Grind and crush the herbs using a mortar and pestle.
3. Moisten with water and make into a thick paste.
4. Apply directly to the skin or place a single layer of gauze bandage against the skin first and apply the poultice to the bandage.
5. Place a dressing or bandage over it to keep it in place.
6. Keep in place for at least 20 minutes but leave it no more than 3 hours before replacing.

Making a Lotion / Cream

Uses:

Lotions and creams are really good to apply to skin conditions and irritations.

Method:

1. Add ½ oz beeswax to 4oz coconut oil.
2. Heat them in a pan until they have melted.
3. Add the selected extract, usually you want to use no more than 20 - 25 drops per mixture.
4. Add to your selected container and leave to cool.

If the consistency is too soft re-melt and add more beeswax.

If the consistency is too hard re-melt and add more coconut oil.

If you don't feel the scent is strong enough you can re-melt and add more of your extract.

Note- you can use essential oils instead of an extract.

Making a Rub / Salve

Uses:

Rubs are really good to apply to chests and areas of inflammation. They can be more convenient than a compress or poultice, especially if you are out and about.

Method:

1. Add 2oz coconut oil to 1oz beeswax.
2. Heat them in a pan until they have melted.
3. Add the selected extracts, usually you want to use no more than 15 - 20 drops per 3oz of mixture.
4. Add to your selected container and leave to cool.

If the consistency is too soft re-melt and add more beeswax.

If the consistency is too hard re-melt and add more coconut oil.

If you don't feel the scent is strong enough you can re-melt and add more of your extract.

Note- you can use essential oils instead of an extract.

Making an Inhalant

Uses:

Inhalants are best used to combat congestion and respiratory complaints.

Method:

1. Fill a glass bowl with boiling water.
2. Add 5-6 drops of herbal extract per ½ pint of water.
3. Place a towel over the bowl and breathe in the vapour.

If you find this method too claustrophobic or feel it makes you cough too much, use a greater quantity of oils, and simply place in the room.

Making a Wash
(USE THE SAME METHOD FOR MAKING A
HERBAL BATH)

Uses:

A wash is generally used as a quick daily treatment and works
best on skin conditions. Use in a bath for aches and pains.

Method:

1. Prepare your washbowl as normal.
2. Add between 3 and 6 drops of herbal extract or
   essential oil to the water. - Increase this quantity for
   baths

Alternatively use a decoction or infusion, using approximately
one cup for a wash and three for a bath.

Herbs: Magical and Medicinal Uses

Using this section

The following section contains a list of herbs and suggested uses.

These suggestions are intended as guidelines, therefore, if something is recommended to be used as a poultice, but you feel a cream or rub would be better suited, then please adapt the information to meet your needs.

Whilst every care has been taken to include appropriate health warnings, if you do suffer from any medical complaints, are taking prescribed medication, or are pregnant or breast feeding, please seek advice from your medicinal practitioner before starting any herbal remedies.

1

Agrimony

Magical attributes: Protection, Sleep, Spell-breaking.

Magical usage:

- Use in Candle magic, Herbal bags, Incense, and Spells.
- Add to a drink or meal to silence those who would tell malicious lies.
- Place in a Herbal bag for protection and place under the pillow to aid with sleep.
- Use in the reversing of a spell.

Medicinal attributes: Antacid, Anti-inflammatory, Astringent, Laxative, Relaxant, Vulnerary.

Medicinal usage:

- A tea made from the leaves can help to reduce acidity in the stomach, as well ease problems affecting the liver, kidney, and spleen.
- Apply poultice of fresh leaves to help heal wounds and reduce varicose veins.
- Bathing in this herb will help to alleviate aches and pains from over exertion.
- Use the cooled tea as a gargle to soothe a sore throat or mouth.
- Use the root to make a tea to help relieve constipation.

2

Alfalfa

Magical attributes: Prosperity.

Magical usage:

- Use in Candle magic, Herbal bags, Incense, and Spells.
- Keep in the home to protect against poverty.
- Place in a Herbal bag and carry with you to protect against being scammed.

Medicinal attributes; Anti-arthritic, Anti-asthmatic, Bitter-tonic, Diuretic.

Medicinal usage:

- Helps to assist in the relief of urinary problems and water retention.
- Use the leaves in cooking or as a tea to improve the appetite.
- Relieves arthritis.

3

Allspice Berries

Magical attributes: Healing, Luck, Prosperity, Success.

Magical usage:

- Use in Candle magic, Herbal bags, Incense, and Spells.
- Use in an incense to attract money.
- Use for all types of healing.

Medicinal attributes: Anaesthetic, Diaphoretic, Relaxant, Rubefacient.

Medicinal usage:

- Apply as a poultice to a specific area to help with poor circulation, stiff joints, and tired muscles.
- Add to a bath for relaxing muscles and promoting healing.

4

Althaea Root (Marshmallow root)

Magical attributes: Attracts Spirits, Healing, Protection.

Magical usage:

- Use in Candle magic, Herbal bags, Incense, and Spells.
- Burn or keep in the home to attract good spirits.
- Carry in Herbal bag for healing and protection.

Medicinal attributes: Anti-inflammatory, Antitussive, Bronchodilator, Expectorant, Vulnerary.

Medicinal usage:

- Apply as poultice to relieve external skin wounds such as boils and abscesses.
- Provides minor relief for urinary tract infections.
- Reduces inflammation and has a calming effect on the body.
- Relieves indigestion and kidney problems.
- Relieves inflammation caused by coughs and colds.
- Use to soothe bronchitis and irritation in the chest due to persistent coughing.

5

Angelica

Magical attributes: Curse-breaking, Draws positive energy, Exorcism, Healing, Hex-breaking, Protection, Repels negative energy, Visions.

Magical usage:

- Use in Candle magic, Herbal bags, Incense, and Spells.
- Add to bath to remove hexes.
- Carry the root in a pouch as a protective talisman.
- Protects against negative energy and attracts positive energy.
- Removes curses, hexes, or spells that have been cast against you.
- Use in exorcism and protection incense.
- Very powerful protection herb.

Medicinal attributes: Abortifacient, Anti-rheumatic, Appetiser, Bitter-tonic, Bronchodilator, Carminative, Diaphoretic, Digestive, Emmenagogue, Expectorant, Tonic.

Medicinal usage:

- Beneficial to the stomach and digestion.
- Gargle for sore throat and mouth.
- Grind the dried root into a powder and apply to athlete's foot.
- Relieves build-up of mucus due to asthma and bronchitis.
- Relieves tension headaches.
- Use as a Poultice for broken bones, itching, rheumatism, and swelling.
- Use as a wash to prevent acne.

Warning - Large doses can negatively affect blood pressure, heart, and respiration.

Warning - Do not use if pregnant.

6

Ashwagandha (Indian Ginseng)

Magical attributes: Energy, Fertility, Health.

Magical usage:

- Use in Candle magic, Herbal bags, Incense, and Spells.
- Drink as a tea before magical practices to boost energy.
- Strengthens Chi energy.
- Use in fertility spells.

Medicinal attributes: Abortifacient, Anti-arthritic, Antidepressant, Anti-inflammatory, Anti-rheumatic, Antitussive, Aphrodisiac, Astringent, Bronchodilator, Carminative, Immunostimulant, Sedative, Tonic.

. . .

Medicinal usage:

- Boosts energy levels, eases chronic fatigue.
- Boosts the immune system.
- Can be used to fight malaria.
- Eases bronchitis and coughs.
- Helps fight depression.
- Helps to build endurance.
- Helps to improve memory and reaction time.
- Promotes restful sleep.
- Reduces anaemia.
- Relieves anxiety and nerves.
- Relieves pain and inflammation of arthritis and rheumatism.

Warning - Do not use if pregnant.

7

Balm

Magical attributes: Healing, Love, Success.

Magical usage:

- Use in Candle magic, Herbal bags, Incense, and Spells.
- Carry to help ease a broken heart.

Medicinal attributes: Anti-asthmatic, Antispasmodic, Bitter-tonic, Bronchodilator, Calmative, Carminative, Diaphoretic, Emmenagogue, Soporific.

Medicinal usage:

- Add an infusion of the leaves to a bath to encourage menstruation.
- Drink as a tea for asthma and bronchitis.
- Drink as a tea for toothache and migraines.
- Drink as a tea to relieve cramps, colic, dyspepsia, flatulence.
- Helps relieve insomnia.
- Helps with nervous problems, hysteria, and melancholy.
- Make into a tea during pregnancy to ease dizziness and headaches.
- Use crushed leaves as a poultice for insect bites, sores, and tumours.

8

Basil

Magical attributes: Exorcism, Fidelity, Love, Prosperity, Protection, Purification, Success.

Magical usage:

- Use in Candle magic, Herbal bags, Incense, and Spells.
- Burn as an exorcism incense.
- Carry to attract wealth.
- Sprinkle on the floor for protection.
- Sprinkle over your sleeping lover to assure fidelity.
- Use in love and prosperity spells.
- Use it in a bath to bring new love in, or to free yourself from an old one.
- Use in purification baths.

Medicinal attributes: Antitussive, Diaphoretic, Digestive, Expectorant, Sedative.

Medicinal usage:

- Drink as a tea after a stressful day to help relaxation.
- Helps relieve coughs and expel mucus from chest, nose, and throat.
- Make as a tea to aid with digestion.

9

Bay Leaves

Magical attributes: Hex-breaking, Purification, Protection, Repels negative energy.

Magical usage:

- Use in Candle magic, Herbal bags, Incense, and Spells.
- Removes unwanted influences, particularly of malevolent intent.
- Sprinkle to cleanse a room.
- Use for Purification, hex-breaking, and protection from evil.
- Use in healing spells.

Medicinal attributes: Anti-nausea, Anti-Rheumatic, Bitter-tonic, Depurative, Sedative.

· · ·

Medicinal usage:

- Apply leaves as a cream or poultice to bruises, skin rashes and sprains.
- Helps to relieve migraine and nausea.
- Purifies the blood.
- Strengthens liver and illnesses affecting the liver.
- Use a rub made from the leaves and apply to rheumatic the aches and pains.

10

Belladonna

Magical attributes: Divination.

Magical usage:

- Use in Candle magic, Herbal bags, Incense, and Spells.

Medicinal attributes: Analgesic, Anti-asthmatic, Antihistamine, Anti-rheumatic, Antispasmodic, Diuretic, Hallucinogenic, Laxative, Sedative.

Medicinal usage:

- Apply as a lotion in case of neuralgia, gout, rheumatism, and sciatica.

- Can be used to treat radiation burns.
- Can help ease problems with the bladder and kidney diseases.
- Helps relieve asthma and whooping cough.
- Helps to relieve irritable bowel syndrome.
- Relieves cold and flu.
- Use as a hay fever remedy.

Warning - Due to its poisonous nature it is very dangerous to use, never use without first seeking a medical opinion.

11

Bilberry

Magical attributes: Protection.

Magical usage:

- Use in Candle magic, Herbal bags, Incense, and Spells.
- Carry bilberry to protect against drowning.

Medicinal attributes: Antiseptic, Astringent, Cardiac.

Medicinal usage:

- Apply as a poultice to relieve haemorrhoids and skin infections.
- Can assist with heart and artery problems.

- Drink as a tea to help gout, kidney problems and urinary tract infection.
- Drink as a tea and apply as a poultice to help fight skin infections.
- Improves eyesight.

Warning - Bilberry leaves can produce symptoms of poisoning if used over long periods.

12

Bitter Melon

Magical attributes: Healing.

Magical usage:

- Use in Candle magic, Herbal bags, Incense, and Spells.

Medicinal attributes: Abortifacient, Anti-rheumatic, Bitter-tonic, Depurative, Emetic, Laxative, Stimulant, Tonic.

Medicinal usage:

- Can cause miscarriage during pregnancy.
- Cools the body.

- Eat the fruit to relieve gout, rheumatism, liver disease, and spleen problems.
- Purifies the blood.

Warning - Do not use if pregnant.

13

Black Snakeroot

Magical attributes: Protection, Strength.

Magical usage:

- Use in Candle magic, Herbal bags, Incense, and Spells.
- Protects and strengthens those who are timid, nervous, or shy.

Medicinal attributes: Anti-arthritic, Antidepressant, Anti-rheumatic, Antitussive, Refrigerant, Vasodilator.

Medicinal usage:

- Apply as poultice or rub to ease arthritis and rheumatism.
- Lowers blood pressure.
- Make a tea to relieve arthritis, depression, dyspepsia, hot flushes, and rheumatism.
- Speeds up recovery after childbirth.

14

Blackberry

Magical attributes: Attracts faeries, Healing, Money, Protection, Repels evil spirits.

Magical usage:

- Use in Candle magic, Herbal bags, Incense, and Spells.
- If added to a wreath with rowan and ivy will keep away evil spirits.
- Powerful herb of protection.
- Use to attract wealth.
- Use to invoke and attract faerie spirits.

Medicinal attributes: Anti-diarrhoea, Astringent, Expectorant, Tonic.

. . .

Medicinal usage:

- Chewing the leaves helps with bleeding gums.
- Eases mucus from nose, throat, and lungs.
- Relieves chronic appendicitis and enteritis leucorrhoea.
- Relieves diarrhoea.

15

Blackcurrant

Magical attributes: Healing, Prophetic dreams, Spirituality, Visions.

Magical usage:

- Use in Candle magic, Herbal bags, Incense, and Spells.
- Eat or drink blackcurrant to aid with prophetic dreams.

Medicinal attributes: Anti-rheumatic, Diaphoretic, Diuretic.

Medicinal usage:

- Blackcurrant juice can help relieve colic.
- Make into a tea for gout and rheumatism.
- The tea when taken cold is also good for throat ailments.
- Use the leaf and berries in a tea to relieve whooping cough.
- Used as a gargle for sore gums.

16

Bladderwrack

Magical attributes: Money, Protection, Psychic abilities, Sea Spells, Wind Spells.

Magical usage:

- Use in Candle magic, Herbal bags, Incense, and Spells.
- Carry when travelling on, or over, water for protection.
- Offers protection to those at sea.
- Use in money spells.
- Use in spells to increase Psychic abilities.
- Wash floors and doors with an infusion to attract positive energy.

Medicinal attributes: Anti-arthritic, Antioxidant, Anti-rheumatic, Antibacterial, Immunostimulant, Laxative.

. . .

Medicinal usage:

- Apply topically to inflamed joints.
- Boosts the immune system.
- Good for healing problems with the Bladder.
- Helps brain development.
- Helps with hair growth.
- Reduces fine lines and wrinkles.
- Regulates an under active thyroid.
- Relieves arthritis and rheumatism.
- Relieves constipation.
- Relieves heartburn.
- Softens and rejuvenates the skin.
- Stops food returning through the oesophagus.
- Treats anaemia.
- Use to relieve urinary tract infections.

17

Blessed Thistle

Magical attributes Protection.

Magical usage:

- Use in Candle magic, Herbal bags, Incense, and Spells.
- Drink as a tea or sprinkle for protection from evil.

Medicinal attributes: Antibacterial, Anti-rheumatic, Bitter-tonic, Expectorant, Galactagogue, Vulnerary.

Medicinal usage:

- Apply as poultice or infusion to treat ulcers and wounds.

- Can help with internal cancers, diabetes, gout, and rheumatism.
- Eat or drink to help with poor appetite, indigestion, flatulence.
- Helps increase milk in nursing mothers.
- Helps to expel excess mucus.
- Use to treat gastrointestinal problems.

18

Blue Cornish Root

Magical attributes: Money, Prosperity, Protection.

Magical usage:

- Use in Candle magic, Herbal bags, Incense, and Spells.
- Used to protect people and places.
- Used in money drawing magic spells for prosperity and wealth.

Medicinal attributes: Abortifacient, Diuretic, Emmenagogue.

Medicinal usage:

- Can cause early period.
- Eases menstrual cramps.
- Helps relieve urinary tract infections.

Warning - Do not use if pregnant.

19

Blue Flag Root

Magical attributes Money, Prosperity.

Magical usage:

- Use in Candle magic, Herbal bags, Incense, and Spells.
- Carry in your purse or wallet to attract money.

Medicinal attributes: Anti-nausea, Bitter-tonic, Diaphoretic, Digestive, Diuretic.

Medicinal usage:

- Aids with digestion and stomach complaints.

- Apply as an extract or infusion to eczema.
- Eases urinary tract infections.
- Relieves migraines.
- Relieves nausea and vomiting.

20

Borage

Magical attributes Courage, Repels evil spirits, Psychic abilities

Magical usage:

- Use in Candle magic, Herbal bags, Incense, and Spells.
- Sprinkle around the house to banish and repel evil.
- Burn as an incense for courage and to increase psychic abilities.

Medicinal attributes: Antipyretic, Carminative, Diaphoretic, Galactagogue, Laxative, Sedative, Tonic.

Medicinal usage:

- Calms and soothes anxiety and nerves.
- Delays male pattern baldness.
- Helps to relieve menstruation symptoms.
- Increases milk in nursing mothers.
- Reduces fevers by drawing out heat.

Warning - Avoid using large amounts and avoid prolonged use.

21

Broom

Magical attributes: Divination, Protection, Purification, Wind Spells.

Magical usage:

- Use in Candle magic, Herbal bags, Incense, and Spells.
- Use in purification baths.
- Sprinkle around the home to purify and protect it.

Medicinal attributes: Cathartic, Diuretic, Emetic.

Medicinal usage:

· · ·

Warning - Very toxic, do not ingest, please look for alternatives with the desired attributes.

22

Burdock

Magical attributes: Healing, Protection.

Magical usage:

- Use in Candle magic, Herbal bags, Incense, and Spells.
- Burn for purification of a room.
- Carry as a protection sachet.
- Used in protection incenses and for healing.

Medicinal attributes: Anti-arthritic, Anti-inflammatory, Anti-rheumatic, Cholagogue, Depurative, Diaphoretic, Diuretic, Laxative, Vulnerary.

Medicinal usage:

- Apply root as a poultice to boils, sores, ulcers, and wounds to promote healing.
- Helps with hair growth.
- Promotes sweating and circulation.
- Purifies the blood.
- Relieves cold and flu.
- Use in a bath, as a poultice and/or ingest to relieve arthritis and rheumatism.

23

Camellia

Magical attributes: Money, Prosperity, Water spells.

Magical usage:

- Use in Candle magic, Herbal bags, Incense, and Spells.
- Place fresh blossoms in water on alter to attract money and prosperity.
- Add to an offering to express gratitude.

Medicinal attributes:

Medicinal usage: Astringent, Tonic.

- Mix with sesame seed oil to treat burns.
- Use as an infusion or poultice to treat skin conditions.

24

Caraway

Magical attributes: Fidelity, Love, Protection, Repels evil spirits.

Magical usage:

- Use in Candle magic, Herbal bags, Incense, and Spells.
- Carry for protection against evil spirits.
- Use in spells to attract a lover.
- Use the seeds to ensure faithfulness.

Medicinal attributes: Anti-arthritic, Anti-nausea, Antipyretic, Anti-rheumatic, Antitussive, Bronchodilator, Carminative, Expectorant.

Medicinal usage:

- Calms anxiety and nerves.
- Eases nausea and vomiting.
- Helps relieve bronchitis, coughs and colds.
- Reduces fevers.
- Relieves arthritis and rheumatism, both by ingestion and application to areas.
- Stops toothache when applied as an extract or infusion to the tooth and gum.
- Treats skin conditions such as acne when applied as an extract or infusion.
- Use as a gargle to relieve a sore throat.

25

Carob

Magical attributes: Exorcism, Prosperity, Protection.

Magical usage:

- Use in Candle magic, Herbal bags, Incense, and Spells.
- Burn as an incense to attract spirit helpers and familiars.
- Burn to deter poltergeists.

Medicinal attributes: Antibacterial, Anti-diarrhoea, Antihistamine, Antitussive, Antiviral, Bitter-tonic, Digestive, Depurative.

Medicinal usage:

- Aids with digestion.
- Can be used to sweeten things.
- Purifies the blood.
- Relieves coughs, colds, and flu.
- Stops diarrhoea.

26

Catnip

Magical attributes: Animal magic, Beauty, Cat magic, Happiness, Love, Psychic abilities, Wishes.

Magical usage:

- Use in Candle magic, Herbal bags, Incense, and Spells.
- Burning the dried leaves for love wishes.
- Increases psychic abilities.
- Increases psychic bond with animals.
- Use during meditation.
- Use for animal magic and healing pets.

Medicinal attributes: Analgesic, Anti-diarrhoea, Antispasmodic, Bronchodilator, Carminative, Diaphoretic.

. . .

Medicinal usage:

- Drink as a tea to soothe and relieve colic, flatulence, spasms, and an upset stomach.
- Helps stop diarrhoea.
- Relieves bronchitis.
- Use as a tea for relaxation.

27

Cayenne Pepper

Magical attributes: Hex-breaking, Fire spells, Love, Power.

Magical usage:

- Use in Candle magic, Herbal bags, Incense, and Spells.
- Adds power to any spell.
- Use in hexes, or to break a hex.
- Use in love or separation spells.

Medicinal attributes: Anti-arthritic, Antispasmodic, Bitter-tonic, Expectorant, Relaxant, Tonic.

Medicinal usage:

- Acts as a digestive aid when taken with food.
- Aids circulation.
- Apply as poultice or rub for joint pain.
- Relieves arthritis
- Relieves colds.
- Use to cleanse wounds.
- Reduces pain of muscle spasms, polyneuropathy, and shingles.
- Relieves headaches, sore throat, and toothache
- Use as an extract or poultice to treat bunions and psoriasis

Warning - Avoid using in large quantities if you suffer from bowel disorders or stomach ulcers.

28

Cedar

Magical attributes: Earth spells, Healing, Love, Money, Protection, Purification.

Magical usage:

- Burn to induce Psychic abilities.
- Burn to purify an area and cure nightmares.
- Keep some in your purse or wallet to attract money.
- Use for grounding.
- Use in Candle magic, Herbal bags, Incense, and Spells.
- Use in money incense.
- Used in love Herbal bags.

Medicinal attributes: Anti-arthritic, Anti-inflammatory, Antiseptic, Anti-rheumatic, Antitussive, Astringent, Diuretic, Emmenagogue, Expectorant, Soporific, Vulnerary.

. . .

Medicinal usage:

- Apply to teeth and gums to relieve toothache.
- Eases itchy skin and psoriasis.
- Promotes a good night sleep.
- Use as a rub on area affected by arthritis or rheumatism to relieve pain and inflammation.
- Use as an extract or poultice on wounds to encourage healing.
- Use as a rub to ease chest complaints, coughs, and colds.

29

Celery Seed

Magical attributes: Prophetic dreams, Psychic abilities.

Magical usage:

- Use in Candle magic, Herbal bags, Incense, and Spells.
- Place under the pillow to help prophetic dreaming.
- Carry to enhance psychic abilities.

Medicinal attributes: Anti-arthritic, Anti-inflammatory, Anti-rheumatic, Antispasmodic, Aphrodisiac, Diuretic, Sedative, Vasodilator

Medicinal usage:

- Drink as a tea to treat urinary tract infection and relieve indigestion.
- Drink, or apply as a rub, to ease and prevent muscle spasms.
- Drink, or apply as a rub, to relieve arthritis and rheumatism.
- Reduces blood pressure.
- Relieves colds.
- Relieves headaches.

30

Chamomile

Magical attributes:, Curse-breaking, Hex-breaking, Love, Money, Prosperity, Purification, Repels the evil eye.

Magical usage:

- Use in Candle magic, Herbal bags, Incense, and Spells.
- Bathe children in it to protect against the evil eye.
- Use in a bath, or to wash your face and hair, to attract love.
- Drink before magic undertakings.
- Use in sleep and meditation incense.
- Use to attract money.
- Useful in breaking curses cast against you.

Medicinal attributes: Analgesic, Antispasmodic, Bitter-tonic, Soporific, Stimulant.

. . .

Medicinal usage:

- Drink before bed to ease insomnia.
- Relieves colic and flatulence.
- Use as a gargle and mouth rinse after having a tooth extracted.
- Use as a rub or tea to ease stomach cramps and spasms.
- Use as a wash for sores and wounds.

31

Cinnamon

Magical attributes: Healing, Love, Luck, Lust, Money, Protection, Psychic abilities, Purification, Spirituality, Success.

Magical usage:

- Use in Candle magic, Herbal bags, Incense, and Spells.
- Burn cinnamon as an incense for healing, money, Psychic abilities, and protection.
- Mix with frankincense, myrrh, and sandalwood for a strong protection incense.

Medicinal attributes: Anti-nausea, Antispasmodic, Bitter-tonic.

Medicinal usage:

- Apply as a liquid or paste to blackheads or spots.
- Good for circulation.
- Helps relieve nausea.
- Helps with stomach upsets and digestive issues.
- Mix with a pinch of cayenne pepper and honey to soothe sore throat.
- Relieves colds and flu.

32

Cloves

Magical attributes: Exorcism, Healing, Luck, Money, Protection, Repels evil spirits, Repels negative energy.

Magical usage:

- Use in Candle magic, Herbal bags, Incense, and Spells.
- Carry for protection.
- Use in incense to attract money, drive away negativity, purify, luck, or to stop gossip.
- Wear or carry for protection or to repel negative energies.
- Make a pomander using cloves, an orange, and a coloured ribbon for a protection or healing charm.

Medicinal attributes: Anaesthetic, Anti-nausea, Antitussive, Anti-asthmatic, Bitter-tonic, Bronchodilator, Expectorant.

Medicinal usage:

- Add clove extract to virgin olive oil and put slightly warmed into the ear for earache.
- Apply as a poultice to ease cramps.
- Apply clove extract to ease toothache or painful gums.
- Chewing a clove with a pinch of salt relieves a sore throat and stops coughs.
- Powdered fried cloves with honey helps stop vomiting.
- Mix clove extract with honey and garlic to relieve tuberculosis, asthma, and bronchitis.
- Rub a clove stalk in water and rub on a stye for relief.

33

Coltsfoot

Magical attributes: Harmony, Love, Peace, Visions.

Magical usage:

- Use in Candle magic, Herbal bags, Incense, and Spells.
- Add to love charms and use in spells for peace and harmony.
- Burning this herb is said to bring visions.

Medicinal attributes: Abortifacient, Anti-asthmatic, Antispasmodic, Antitussive, Astringent, Bronchodilator, Demulcent, Emollient, Expectorant.

Medicinal usage:

- Soothes sore throat and coughs.
- Helps to relieve bronchitis.
- Treats bronchitis, whooping cough, asthma, and chronic emphysema.

Warning - Do not use if pregnant or nursing.

34

Comfrey

Magical attributes:, Astral Projection, Money, Protection, Repels negative energy, Travel safety.

Magical usage:

- Use in Candle magic, Herbal bags, Incense, and Spells.
- A strong herb for protection against any type of negativity.
- Especially good for protection while travelling.
- Protection in the astral realms.

Medicinal attributes: Analgesic, Astringent, Demulcent, Emollient, Expectorant, Astringent, Refrigerant, Sedative, Vulnerary, Anti-diarrhoea

. . .

Medicinal usage:

.

- Apply as extract or poultice to blemishes and scars to reduce visibility.
- Drink as a tea to help ease diarrhoea.
- Helps to heal fractures and sprains.
- Use as a gargle to treat bleeding gums and sore throat.
- Wash with an infusion to help treat eczema and psoriasis.

35

Country Mallow (Indian Mallow)

Magical attributes: Healing, Repels negative energy.

Magical usage:

- Use in Candle magic, Herbal bags, Incense, and Spells.
- Bathe in an infusion to repel and rid yourself of negative feelings.
- Place around the home to protect the home from negative energy.

Medicinal attributes: Analgesic, Anti-arthritic, Anti-inflammatory, Antipyretic, Anti-rheumatic, Carminative, Diaphoretic, Diuretic, Relaxant, Tonic, Vasodilator.

Medicinal usage:

- Apply as an extract to ease sore joints and muscles.
- Drink, and apply as rub, to ease pain and inflammation of arthritis and rheumatism.
- Drink as a tea to relieve anxiety and nervous disorders.
- Eases rheumatism.
- Lowers the blood pressure.
- Reduces fevers.
- Relieves colic.
- Use the root to treat facial paralysis and sciatica.
- Use a decoction for toothache and sore gums.
- Apply as an extract or poultice to boils and ulcers.

36

Cowslip

Magical attributes: Healing, Repels evil spirits, Youth

Magical usage:

- Use in Candle magic, Herbal bags, Incense, and Spells.
- Burn to repel evil spirits.

Medicinal attributes: Analgesic, Anti-arthritic, Anti-rheumatic, Antispasmodic, Antitussive, Diaphoretic, Diuretic, Expectorant, Rubefacient

Medicinal usage:

- Apply as extract, or wash in infusion, to reduce blemishes and spots.
- Eases arthritis and rheumatism.
- Eases coughs.
- Strengthens nerves.
- Use as a wash to revive the skin and reduce fine lines and wrinkles.
- Drink as a tea to relieve urinary tract infections.

37

Cumin

Magical attributes: Repels evil spirits, Love, Protection.

Magical usage:

- Use in Candle magic, Herbal bags, Incense, and Spells.
- Burn with frankincense for protection.
- Mix with salt and sprinkle to keep away evil spirits and bad luck.
- Use in love spells.

Medicinal attributes: Anti-diarrhoea, Anti-nausea, Antitussive, Sedative

Medicinal usage:

- Drink to relieve cold and fevers.
- Eases morning sickness.
- Helps treat colic and flatulence.
- Eases diarrhoea if mixed as 1tsp of cumin seed to 1tsp of coriander with a pinch of salt and drank as a tea after eating.
- Use as a gargle for a sore throat.

38

Custard Apple

Magical attributes: Healing.

Magical usage:

- Use in Candle magic, Herbal bags, Incense, and Spells.

Medicinal attributes: Abortifacient, Anti-diarrhoea, Bitter-tonic, Expectorant, Sedative, Tonic.

Medicinal usage:

- Drink a tea made from the leaves to relieve cold.
- Drink a tea made from the root to ease diarrhoea.

- Drink as a tea to ease urinary tract infections.
- Strengthens the digestive system.
- Use the leaves to overcome hysteria and fainting spells.

Warning - Do not use if pregnant.

39

Damiana

Magical attributes: Lust, Love, Visions

Magical usage:

- Use in Candle magic, Herbal bags, Incense, and Spells.
- Burn to enhance visions.
- Use in lust and love spells.

Medicinal attributes: Antidepressant, Aphrodisiac, Carminative, Relaxant Stimulant, Vasodilator.

Medicinal usage:

- Aids people suffering from mild depression.

- Calms anxiety and the nerves.
- Consume as an aphrodisiac.
- Drink as a tea to relieve a hangover.
- Drink as a tea to treat anxiety, exhaustion, and nerves.
- Helps to treat and ease menopausal problems, painful menstruation, prostate complaints, and urinary tract infections.
- Lifts the spirits.
- Regulates hormones.

40

Dandelion

Magical attributes: Attracts Spirits, Divination, Healing, Protection, Psychic abilities.

Magical usage:

- Use in Candle magic, Herbal bags, Incense, and Spells.
- Burn to attract spirits.
- Drink the root as a tea to enhance Psychic abilities.
- Use in healing and protection spells.
- Use in Samhain rituals.
- Use the flowers and leaves in a tea for healing.

Medicinal attributes: Anti-asthmatic, Anti-arthritic, Anti-rheumatic, Bitter-tonic, Cholagogue, Diuretic, Tonic.

• • •

Medicinal usage:

- Apply fresh sap for several weeks to remove a wart.
- As a tea it can ease asthma, bone problems, gout, and swollen glands.
- Drink as a tea to help eliminate gall and kidney stones.
- Helps ease arthritis and rheumatism.
- Helps remove toxins from the body.
- Use as a gargle to help with bad breath and mouth ulcers.
- Wash with a dandelion infusion to treat eczema and other skin conditions.

41

Dill

Magical attributes: Anti-hex, Lust, Love, Money, Protection.

Magical usage:

- Use in Candle magic, Herbal bags, Incense, and Spells.
- Carry for protection.
- Hang in the doorway to protect your home.
- Use in love and lust spells.
- Use in money spells.

Medicinal attributes: Anti-arthritic, Antibacterial, Anti-diarrhoea, Anti-rheumatic, Bitter-tonic, Carminative, Immunostimulant, Stimulant.

. . .

Medicinal usage:

- Boosts immune system.
- Can help relieve diarrhoea.
- Dill is said to "destroyeth the hiccups"*
- Eases flatulence.
- Relieves arthritis and rheumatism.

*source: http://www.bristolbotanicals.co.uk

42

Elder Flower

Magical attributes: Anti-Theft, Healing, Prosperity, Protection, Repels negative energy.

Magical usage:

- Use in Candle magic, Herbal bags, Incense, and Spells.
- Sprinkle for protection from criminals and from the law.

Medicinal attributes: Antihistamine, Anti-inflammatory, Antioxidant, Antiviral, Diaphoretic, Diuretic, Expectorant, Laxative, Emollient

Medicinal usage:

- Apply the bark as a poultice on minor burns and chilblains.
- Bathe sore eyes, irritated and inflamed skin, and minor wounds in an infusion.
- Drink as a tea to ease fevers, hay fever, respiratory complaints, and sinusitis.
- Drink as a tea to treat colds and flu.
- The fruit helps to relieve constipation.
- Use as a gargle to ease mouth ulcers.

43

Elecampane

Magical attributes: Love, Repels negative energy.

Magical usage:

- Use in Candle magic, Herbal bags, Incense, and Spells.
- Use Elecampane, Mistletoe, and Verbena to create a medieval true love powder.
- Sprinkle around the threshold to keep negative energies and influences at bay.

Medicinal attributes: Anti-asthmatic, Antidepressant, Antitussive, Bronchodilator, Depurative, Expectorant, Vulnerary.

Medicinal usage:

- Apply as an extract or poultice to wounds to ease pain.
- Apply topically to treat skin conditions, psoriasis, scabies, and herpes.
- Helps relieve asthma, bronchitis, emphysema, and whooping cough.
- Helps to clear rubbish from nose, throat, and chest.
- Helps ward off depression.
- Purifies the blood.
- Relieves symptoms of a cold.

44

Eucalyptus Leaf

Magical attributes: Draws positive energy, Healing, Protection, Purification.

Magical usage:

- Use in Candle magic, Herbal bags, Incense, and Spells.
- Attracts healing vibrations and protection.
- Use in a purification or healing bath.
- Use to purify and cleanse any space of unwanted energies.

Medicinal attributes: Anti-arthritic, Anti-asthmatic, Antibacterial, Antifungal, Anti-rheumatic, Antiseptic, Antitussive, Antiviral, Decongestant, Expectorant, Immunostimulant.

. . .

Medicinal usage:

- Apply as a rub to areas suffering with arthritis, rheumatism, or nerve pain for relief.
- Apply as extract or rub to chest to relieve coughs and ease congestion.
- Bathe wounds in it to promote healing and fight infections.
- Boosts the immune system.
- Expels mucus from lungs, nose, and throat, relieving congestion.
- Kills germs and fights infections.
- Treats colds, congestion, coughs, flu, and sinusitis.

45

Eyebright

Magical attributes: Mental powers, Psychic abilities.

Magical usage:

- Use in Candle magic, Herbal bags, Incense, and Spells.
- Carry to increase psychic abilities.

Medicinal attributes: Astringent, Tonic.

Medicinal usage:

- Apply a poultice of the leaves to eyes to soothe them.
- Bathe infected, tired, or sores eyes in an infusion.

- Drink a tea to revitalise and strengthen the body.
- Used for all manner of eye complaints.
- Apply to a stye to ease inflammation and soreness.

46

Fennel Seed

Magical attributes: Anti-curse, Courage, Healing, Longevity, Protection, Purification, Strength, Vitality.

Magical usage:

- Use in Candle magic, Herbal bags, Incense, and Spells.
- Prevents curses, possession, and negativity.
- Use for protection spells.
- Use for purification.

Medicinal attributes: Anti-diarrhoea, Anti-nausea, Antispasmodic, Bitter-tonic, Carminative, Digestive, Diuretic, Expectorant, Galactagogue, Stimulant.

Medicinal usage:

- Aids digestion.
- Eases flatulence, colic, irritable bowel syndrome, and stomach cramps.
- Helps stop diarrhoea and ease constipation.
- Helps relieve nausea and vomiting.
- Use as a gargle to help with bad breath.

47

Feverfew

Magical attributes: Healing, Love, Protection, Travel safety.

Magical usage:

- Use in Candle magic, Herbal bags, Incense, and Spells.
- A strong herb for health and spiritual healing.
- Protects travellers, keep in your bag or vehicle when travelling.
- Use to ward off sickness and boost the immune system.

Medicinal attributes: Anti-arthritic, Anti-nausea, Anti-rheumatic, Antispasmodic, Immunostimulant, Carminative.

. . .

Medicinal usage:

- Apply as a cream, extract, or infusion to ease skin conditions, eczema, and psoriasis.
- Eases nausea.
- Eases painful menstruation.
- Excellent treatment for migraine headaches.
- Helps calm nerves and ease anxiety.
- Helps relieve cold and flu.
- Reduces pain of arthritis, rheumatism, and muscle spasms.
- Relieves colic and flatulence.

48

Flaxseed

Magical attributes: Absorbs negative energy, Beauty, Healing, Money, Peace, Protection, Psychic abilities.

Magical usage:

- Use in Candle magic, Herbal bags, Incense, and Spells.
- Carry to attract money.
- Place in a bowl to absorb negative energy.
- Use in healing and protection spells.
- Use to keep the peace at home.

Medicinal attributes: Anti-arthritic, Antidepressant, Anti-diarrhoea, Anti-rheumatic, Antitussive, Bitter-tonic, Demulcent, Digestive, Emollient, Purgative.

. . .

Medicinal usage:

- A decoction can be used for coughs and catarrh.
- Aids with digestion.
- Eases depression.
- Eating the seed relieves constipation.
- Relieves diarrhoea.
- Relieves urinary tract infections.
- Use as a poultice to ease arthritis and rheumatic pain.

49

Fumitory

Magical attributes: Exorcism, Money, Purification.

Magical usage:

- Use in Candle magic, Herbal bags, Incense, and Spells.
- Use with sage to purify a new home.

Medicinal attributes: Anti-diarrhoea, Bitter-tonic, Cholagogue, Diuretic, Laxative, Tonic.

Medicinal usage:

- Drink as a tea for liver and gallbladder problems.

- Drink or eat for scabies and other skin problems.
- Take in large doses for laxative effects but excessive doses can cause diarrhoea and stomach-ache.
- Use as a cream or wash on skin conditions and eczema.

50

Galangal Root

Magical attributes: Courage, Curse-breaking, Helps avoid legal problems, Luck, Money, Psychic abilities, Strength.

Magical usage:

- Use in Candle magic, Herbal bags, Incense, and Spells.
- Burn to break spells and remove curses.
- Place in leather with something silver to attract money.
- Wear or carry for good luck and protection.
- Wear as a talisman for health.

Medicinal attributes: Antibacterial, Anti-nausea, Antispasmodic, Antipyretic, Antitussive, Bitter, Bitter-tonic, Bronchodilator, Carminative, Digestive.

. . .

Medicinal usage:

- Calms anxiety and nerves.
- Eases bronchitis and coughs.
- Eases nausea.
- Promotes digestion.
- Reduces fevers by drawing out heat.
- Use as a gargle for bad breath, bleeding gums, and mouth ulcers.

51

Garlic

Magical attributes: Anti-Theft, Exorcism, Healing, Protection, Lust.

Magical usage:

- Use in Candle magic, Herbal bags, Incense, and Spells.
- Use in protection spells.

Medicinal attributes: Anti-asthmatic, Antibiotic, Antifungal, Antihistamine, Antipyretic, Antispasmodic, Antiviral, Bronchodilator, Carminative, Cholagogue, Depurative, Digestive, Diuretic, Expectorant, Tonic.

Medicinal usage:

- Cleanses the kidneys.
- Fights infections.
- For earache add extract to warmed virgin olive oil and apply to ear canal.
- Purifies the blood.
- Relieves asthma and bronchitis.
- Relieves hay fever and allergies.
- Strengthens body.
- Strong healing properties.

52

Ginger

Magical attributes: Love, Money, Power, Success.

Magical usage:

- Use in Candle magic, Herbal bags, Incense, and Spells.
- Eating before performing spells increases their power
- Use in love spells.

Medicinal attributes: Anti-arthritic, Anti-diarrhoea, Anti-inflammatory, Anti-nausea, Anti-rheumatic, Antitussive, Bitter-tonic, Expectorant.

Medicinal usage:

- A good pain killer.
- Apply to soothe and treat minor burns, eczema, inflammation, and psoriasis.
- Boosts the immune system.
- Calms the stomach.
- Drink as a tea to relieve a fever.
- Eases arthritis, rheumatism, and joint pain.
- Eases coughs and colds.
- Eases indigestion.
- Helps stop diarrhoea.
- Reduces fever.
- Relieves headaches.
- Relieves nausea and vomiting.

53

Ginseng

Magical attributes: Beauty, Curse-breaking, Health, Hex-breaking, Love, Money, Repels evil spirits.

Magical usage:

- Use in Candle magic, Herbal bags, Incense, and Spells.
- Burn to break curses or ward off evil spirits.
- Carry to enhance beauty.
- Use the root in spells for health, love, and money.

Medicinal attributes: Antidepressant, Bitter-tonic, Immunostimulant, Digestive.

Medicinal usage:

- Aids digestion.
- American ginseng can protect against colds and reduce their symptoms.
- Boosts the immune system.
- Can help relieve depression.
- Improves concentration.

54

Goat's Rue

Magical attributes: Anti-curse, Anti-hex, Anti-spell, Healing, Health, Repels the evil eye.

Magical usage:

- Use in Candle magic, Herbal bags, Incense, and Spells.
- Use as an incense to prevent illness
- Wear to ward off the evil eye.
- Defends against harmful spells.

Medicinal attributes: Antidote, Depurative, Diaphoretic, Digestive, Diuretic, Galactagogue.

Medicinal usage:

- Aid with digestion.
- Increases milk in nursing mothers.
- Purifies the blood.
- Use on bites from poisonous animals.

55

Goldenrod

Magical attributes: Divination, Money.

Magical usage:

- Use in Candle magic, Herbal bags, Incense, and Spells.
- Drink as a tea to enhance divination abilities.
- Place in purse to draw money.

Medicinal attributes: Anti-arthritic, Anti-diarrhoea, Antihistamine, Antitussive, Astringent, Bronchodilator, Diuretic, Vulnerary.

Medicinal usage:

- Can help to pass kidney and gall bladder stones.
- Drink as a tea and wash in an infusion for chronic eczema and skin conditions.
- Drink as a tea for arthritis, nephritis, and whooping cough.
- Effective against bronchitis, colds, laryngitis, pneumonia, and sore throat.
- Helps stop diarrhoea.
- Helps to flush the kidneys.
- Relieves symptoms of hay fever.
- Use as a gargle for sore throat.
- Use the fresh leaves as a poultice to relieve insect bites, sores, and wounds.

56

Heather

Magical attributes: Rain magic, Luck, Peace, Protection.

Magical usage:

- Use in Candle magic, Herbal bags, Incense, and Spells.
- Burn during rain magic.
- Carry to protect yourself against violence.
- Hang in the home to bring peace.

Medicinal attributes: Antiseptic, Anti-rheumatic, Antitussive, Cholagogue, Diaphoretic, Diuretic, Expectorant, Sedative, Soporific, Vasoconstrictor.

Medicinal usage:

- Bathe skin conditions in an infusion to treat and relieve irritation.
- Drink to improve skin conditions
- Eases gout and rheumatic pain.
- Helps relieve insomnia.
- Relieves stomach-ache and coughs.

57

Henna

Magical attributes: Healing, Love, Repels the evil eye.

Magical usage:

- Use in Candle magic, Herbal bags, Incense, and Spells.
- Applying henna to the forehead will relieve a headache and protect the third eye.
- Wear in a talisman to attract love.

Medicinal attributes: Abortifacient, Anti-inflammatory, Antipyretic, Antitussive, Astringent, Bitter, Bronchodilator, Decongestant, Depurative, Diuretic, Emmenagogue, Emollient, Expectorant, Refrigerant, Soporific, Vulnerary.

Medicinal usage:

- Apply leaves as a poultice to wounds and ulcers.
- Bathe irritated skin in an infusion to draw out the heat.
- Helps expel mucus and ease congestion.
- Helps promote sleep.
- Helps to ease bronchitis.
- Purifies the blood.
- Relieves coughs and colds.
- Soothes headaches and fevers.
- Use as an infusion to treat wounds.

Warning - Do not use if pregnant.

58

Hibiscus Flower

Magical attributes: Love, Psychic abilities.

Magical usage:

- Enhance psychic ability and divination.
- Use in Candle magic, Herbal bags, Incense, and Spells.
- Use in love spells.
- Use to induce dreams.

Medicinal attributes: Anti-inflammatory, Antispasmodic, Astringent, Bitter-tonic, Carminative, Digestive, Diuretic, Laxative.

Medicinal usage:

- Bathe allergenic eczema in an infusion.
- Bathe itchy skin with an infusion to reduce irritation.
- Drink as a tea to aid digestion.
- Drinking as a tea helps relieve colds, mucus in the nose, throat, and chest.
- Helps ease anxiety and nerves.
- Promotes a healthy appetite.
- Use as a gargle to help bad breath.

59

Holly Leaf

Magical attributes: Dream magic, Luck, Protection.

Magical usage:

- Use in Candle magic, Herbal bags, Incense, and Spells.
- A powerful protective herb.
- Repels poison, evil spirits, and other harmful forces.
- Use the wood to craft magical tools to enhance your intention.

Medicinal attributes: Anti-arthritic, Anti-rheumatic, Diuretic.

Medicinal usage:

- A tea made from dried holly leaves can treat arthritis, gout, rheumatism, and urinary tract infections.
- Juice from fresh leaves can help with jaundice.

Warning - Berries are toxic,

_____

_____

60

Hops

_____

Magical attributes: Energy, Healing, Mental focus, Sleep.

Magical usage:

- Use in Candle magic, Herbal bags, Incense, and Spells.
- Burn during healing prayers.
- Drink as a tea after magical practices to balance your energy.
- Put inside pillow to induce sleep.
- Use in healing charms.
- Use in healing incenses and spells.

Medicinal attributes: Antibiotic, Bitter-tonic, Bronchodilator, Carminative, Sedative, Soporific.

. . .

Medicinal usage:

- Bathe in an infusion to heal and soothe eczema, ulcers, rashes, dry or cracked skin, bruises and other wounds.
- Drink as a tea or use as a gargle for a sore throat.
- Drink as a tea to calm anxiety and nerves.
- Drink as a tea to relieve insomnia.
- Fights infections.
- Helps ease coughs brought on by nerves or tension.
- Helps relieve bronchitis and high fevers.
- Helps to soothe toothache and earache.
- Quickens healing of skin conditions.

61

Horehound

Magical attributes: Energy, Mental focus, Protection, Repels negative energy, Strength, Wishes.

Magical usage:

- Use in Candle magic, Herbal bags, Incense, and Spells.
- Burn for protection wishes.
- Drink as a tea to aid concentration, energy, and focus.
- Tie flowering horehound with a black ribbon and hang in your home for protection against negative energy.
- Use to bless your home.

Medicinal   attributes: Anti-asthmatic,   Anti-nausea,
Antitussive,   Bitter-tonic,   Bronchodilator,   Diaphoretic,
Digestive, Diuretic, Expectorant, Stimulant, Tonic.

Medicinal usage:

- Apply as a poultice to animal bites.
- Apply to skin irritations as a poultice, or wash with an infusion.
- Eases menstrual cramp and helps regulate menstruation.
- Helps stop nausea and vomiting.
- Promotes digestion.
- Soothes dry coughs.
- Use as an infusion to bathe abrasions, eczema, shingles, and wounds.
- Use to ease asthma, bronchitis, coughs, colds, earache, sinusitis, and sore throat.

62

Hyssop

Magical attributes: Purification, Protection

Magical usage:

- Use in Candle magic, Herbal bags, Incense, and Spells.
- An excellent purifying herb.
- Physical and spiritual protection.
- Use in purification baths and spells.

Medicinal attributes: Anti-inflammatory, Antitussive, Astringent, Bitter-tonic, Carminative, Digestive, Emmenagogue, Expectorant, Stimulant, Tonic, Vulnerary.

Medicinal usage:

- Apply a poultice of the crushed leaves to bruises and wounds to cure infection and assist healing.
- Drink as a tea to aid digestion.
- Eases and treats flatulence and jaundice.
- Helps ease coughs, colds, and nose and throat infections.
- Use as a decoction to relieve inflammation.
- Use as a gargle for catarrh and sore throat.
- Uses as an infusion to treat burns, bruises, and skin irritations.

63

Indian Rose Chestnut

Magical attributes: Love, Protection.

Magical usage:

- Use in Candle magic, Herbal bags, Incense, and Spells.
- Bathe in the flowers to attract love.

Medicinal attributes: Abortifacient, Analgesic, Anti-asthmatic, Anti-nausea, Anti-rheumatic, Astringent, Antitussive, Bitter-tonic, Depurative.

Medicinal usage:

- Apply an extract of the seed to skin conditions.

- Apply an infusion from dried flowers to bleeding haemorrhoids.
- Apply an infusion made from fresh flowers to external itchy areas and piles.
- Apply extract from the seeds to rheumatism, sores, scabies, and wounds.
- Drink a tea from fresh flowers to relieve nausea.
- Eases asthma.
- Relieves coughs and colds.

Warning - Do not use if pregnant.

64

Irish Moss

Magical attributes: Luck, Money, Protection.

Magical usage:

- Use in Candle magic, Herbal bags, Incense, and Spells.
- Carry in your purse or wallet to attract money.

Medicinal attributes: Anti-diarrhoea, Antitussive, Antiviral, Bronchodilator, Demulcent, Expectorant.

Medicinal usage:

- Apply as a cream, or wash, to dermatitis, dry and chapped skin eczema, psoriasis, rashes, and sunburn.

- Apply topically to reduce dark circles under the eyes and to keep skin soft and smooth.
- Drink as a tea to treat bronchitis, coughs, pneumonia, respiratory infections, and tuberculosis.
- Eases a hangover.
- Helps stop diarrhoea.
- Helps to treat viral infections.
- Reduces fine lines and wrinkles.

65

Jasmine Flowers

Magical attributes: Love, Psychic dreams.

Magical usage:

- Use in Candle magic, Herbal bags, Incense, and Spells.
- Bathe with jasmine flowers to attract love.
- Drink as a tea or place around your bed to aids in reception of psychic dreams.

Medicinal attributes: Analgesic, Antidepressant, Antiseptic, Aphrodisiac, Astringent, Galactagogue, Carminative, Refrigerant, Sedative.

Medicinal usage:

- Drink as a tea to treat fevers and infections.
- Increases milk production in nursing mothers.
- Relieves anxiety and nerves.
- Use as an extract to ease depression.
- Use as an extract to treat wounds.

66

Juniper Berry

Magical attributes: Anti-Theft, Draws positive energy, Exorcism, Health, Love, Protection, Psychic abilities, Repels negative energy.

Magical usage:

- Use in Candle magic, Herbal bags, Incense, and Spells.
- Anoint an item with the extract to protect from theft.
- Attracts good energies and love.
- Burn for protection.
- Burn or carry to enhance Psychic abilities.
- Use for all kinds of protection magic.
- Repels negative energy.

Medicinal attributes: Anti-arthritic, Anti-rheumatic, Antiseptic, Bitter-tonic, Depurative, Diuretic, Vulnerary, Digestive, Carminative

Medicinal usage:

- Aids in relief of intestinal cramps and treats urinary tract infections.
- Apply to teeth and gums to ease toothache.
- Drink as a tea to relieve the pain of arthritis, rheumatism, and gout.
- Eases colic, dyspepsia, and flatulence.
- Helps with digestion.
- Purifies the blood.
- Relieves anxiety, mental exhaustion, nervous tension, and stress.
- Use as a cream or poultice on athlete's foot, eczema, psoriasis, and slow healing wounds.
- Use the berries topically to ease arthritis, neuralgia, and rheumatism.

67

Ladies Mantle

Magical attributes: Beauty, Fertility, Love, Protection.

Magical usage:

- Use in Candle magic, Herbal bags, Incense, and Spells.
- Place under the bed when trying to conceive.
- Use in a bath to enhance beauty.

Medicinal attributes: Anti-diarrhoea, Antiseptic, Astringent, Febrifuge, Tonic, Vulnerary.

Medicinal usage:

- Eases stomach complaints and menstrual problems.

- Improves appetite.
- Use as a gargle after having a tooth extracted.
- Use as a gargle for sore mouth and ulcers.
- Use as a wash or poultice for wounds.
- Use as a wash to rejuvenate skin.

68

Lavender

Magical attributes: Friendship, Happiness, Longevity, Love, Peace, Protection, Purification, Sleep.

Magical usage:

- Use in Candle magic, Herbal bags, Incense, and Spells.
- Hang in the home for protection.
- Place under the pillow to aid with sleep.
- Use in a bath to promote happiness, love, and peace.

Medicinal attributes: Antidepressant, Anti-nausea, Antiseptic, Antispasmodic, Bitter-tonic, Carminative, Cholagogue, Diuretic, Sedative, Soporific, Stimulant, Tonic, Vulnerary.

. . .

Medicinal usage:

- Apply leaves as a poultice to burns, cuts, and minor wounds.
- Eases nausea, stomach problems, and vomiting.
- Helps ease symptoms of premenstrual syndrome.
- Helps to relieve anxiety, depression, and insomnia.
- Relieves flatulence, migraine headache, fainting, and dizziness.

69

Lemon Grass

Magical attributes: Love, Protection, Psychic abilities.

Magical usage:

- Use in Candle magic, Herbal bags, Incense, and Spells.
- Add to an amulet or charm to increase its power.

Medicinal attributes: Analgesic, Anti-arthritic, Antifungal, Antioxidant, Antipyretic, Antitussive, Antiviral, Bitter-tonic, Immunostimulant, Refrigerant, Sedative.

Medicinal usage:

- Boosts the immune system.

- Eases arthritic pains and sports injuries.
- Eases coughs, colds, and flu.
- Reduces fevers.
- Relieves flatulence, painful menstruation, and gastric irritability.
- Treats viral infections.
- Using as a wash can reduce eczema and spots.

70

Lungwort

Magical attributes: Earth spells, Healing, Sympathetic magic.

Magical usage:

- Use in Candle magic, Herbal bags, Incense, and Spells.
- Powerful healing herb.
- Very effective in sympathetic magic healing.

Medicinal attributes: Anti-asthmatic, Anti-diarrhoea, Antitussive, Astringent, Bronchodilator, Demulcent, Emollient, Expectorant.

Medicinal usage:

- Drink as a tea to relieve diarrhoea.
- Effective against asthma, bronchitis, coughs, and tuberculosis.
- Use as a wash or dressing for haemorrhoids and wounds.

71

Mandrake Root

Magical attributes: Courage, Curse-breaking, Hex-breaking, Fertility, Health, Love, Money, Power, Prosperity, Protection.

Magical usage:

- Use in Candle magic, Herbal bags, Incense, and Spells.
- Burn it or bathe in it to break curses, hexes, and jinxes.
- Carry to attract love and courage.
- Place a whole root in your home for protection and prosperity.
- Place under the bed when trying to conceive.

Medicinal attributes: Anaesthetic, Aphrodisiac.

• • •

Medicinal usage:

Due to its poisonous nature, please refer to other herbs with the desired attributes.

Warning - poisonous, do not ingest.

72

Meadowsweet

Magical attributes: Divination, Happiness Love, Peace, Purification, Water spells.

Magical usage:

- Use in Candle magic, Herbal bags, Incense, and Spells.
- Add to magical tools when casting love spells or rites to increase potency.
- Inhale the scent each night to help find your soulmate.
- Place on altar when making love charms.
- Use in purification baths and rituals.
- Use in water spells to enhance power.

Medicinal attributes: Anti-arthritic, Anti-diarrhoea, Anti-rheumatic, Astringent, Bronchodilator, Diaphoretic, Diuretic, Expectorant.

Medicinal usage:

- Apply as a wash to sore eyes and wounds.
- Drink as a tea for bladder and kidney ailments.
- Helps relieve arthritis, fever, gout, and rheumatism.
- Relieves diarrhoea.
- Use to relieve bronchitis, colds, flu, and respiratory problems.

73

Milkweed

Magical attributes: Attracts faeries, Attracts Spirits, Divination, Protection, Wishes.

Magical usage:

- Use in Candle magic, Herbal bags, Incense, and Spells.
- Burn to add power to wishes.
- Carry for protection.
- Plant in the garden to attract faeries and nature spirits.

Medicinal attributes: Abortifacient, Anti-arthritic, Anti-asthmatic, Anti-inflammatory, Antipyretic, Bronchodilator, Depurative, Expectorant, Laxative, Tonic.

· · ·

Medicinal usage:

- Apply the fresh juice to warts for several weeks.
- Drink as a tea for kidney complaints and stomach problems.
- Eases the pain and inflammation of arthritis.
- Reduces inflammation.
- The flowers help relieve asthma and catarrh.
- The root helps ease asthma, bronchitis, and dyspepsia.
- Use leaves in treatment of arthralgia, fever, paralysis, and swelling.

Warning - Do not use if pregnant.

74

Mint (Mentha)

Magical attributes: Jinx-breaking, Curse-breaking, Hex-breaking, Spell-breaking, Healing, Protection, Psychic abilities, Strength.

Magical usage:

- Use in Candle magic, Herbal bags, Incense, and Spells.
- Carry for protection.
- Drink as a tea to increase psychic abilities
- Use in breaking curses, hexes, jinxes, and spells.
- Use in healing spells or rites.

Medicinal attributes: Anti-nausea, Antioxidant, Bitter-tonic, Carminative, Decongestant, Sedative.

. . .

Medicinal usage:

- Calms anxiety and soothes nerves.
- Fights bad breath.
- Helps relieve congestion from nose, throat, and chest.
- Relieve symptoms of indigestion, heartburn, and irritable bowel syndrome.
- Relieves chest and respiratory system.
- Relieves the symptoms of colds and flu.
- Soothes stomach complaints, nausea, and vomiting.
- Use as an extract or wash and apply to eczema, itchy skin, and minor burns.
- Use to ease nasal allergies.
- Use as an extract or rub to ease aches and pains, cramps, and sprains.

75

Mistletoe

Magical attributes:, Beauty, Exorcism, Fertility, Health, Love, Protection.

Magical usage:

- Use in Candle magic, Herbal bags, Incense, and Spells.
- Burn to drive away unwanted spirits.
- Carry for beauty and protection.
- Hang near the threshold to attract love.
- Place over the bed, or bedroom door to repel nightmares.
- Use Elecampane, Mistletoe, and Verbena to create a medieval true love powder.

Medicinal attributes: Anti-arthritic, Cardiac, Digestive, Diuretic, Immunostimulant, Stimulant, Vasodilator.

. . .

Medicinal usage:

- Aids with digestion.
- Apply as poultice or compress to varicose veins.
- Boosts the immune system.
- Helps to treat and reduce symptoms of arthritis, epilepsy, and menopause.
- Relieves headaches.
- Use to wash chilblains and leg ulcers.

76

Morning Glory Blossoms

Magical attributes: Astral Projection, Divination, Happiness, Peace, Psychic dreams, Visions.

Magical usage:

- Use in Candle magic, Herbal bags, Incense, and Spells.
- Place under your pillow to stop nightmares and assist with psychic dreams.
- Use the vines in binding spells.
- Wear or have on you during astral travel.

Medicinal attributes: Laxative.

Medicinal usage:

- The seeds can be used as a laxative.

Warning - Toxic. Do not consume without medical approval.

77

Moss

Magical attributes: Earth spells, Luck, Money, Prosperity.

Magical usage:

- Use in Candle magic, Herbal bags, Incense, and Spells.
- Use for Gnome magic and earth spells.
- Use in luck spells.
- Use in prosperity spells.

Medicinal attributes: Absorbent.

Medicinal usage:

- Sphagnum moss can be used as a dressing for a bleeding wound instead of a cotton dressing.

Mugwort

Magical attributes: Astral Projection, Divination, Dragon magic, Healing, Prophetic dreams, Protection, Purification, Psychic abilities, Strength.

Magical usage:

- Use in Candle magic, Herbal bags, Incense, and Spells.
- Burn with sandalwood in divination and scrying rituals.
- Drink as a tea sweetened with honey before divination.
- Wear of have on you during astral travel.
- Place leaves on your altar or around you to aid with scrying.
- Place under your pillow for prophetic dreams.
- Used to wash crystal balls and magic mirrors.

Medicinal attributes: Abortifacient, Anti-arthritic, Antidepressant, Anti-rheumatic, Appetiser, Bitter-tonic, Cholagogue, Digestive, Relaxant, Purgative.

Medicinal usage:

- Helps to ease depression and fatigue.
- Aids with appetite and digestion.
- Use an infusion in the bath to relieve aching muscles, arthritis, gout, and rheumatism.
- Apply fresh sap to relieve itching caused by poison oak.

Warning - Do not use if pregnant.

Warning - Large doses can cause symptoms of poisoning.

79

Mullein

Magical attributes: Attracts Spirits, Courage, Divination, Exorcism, Protection.

Magical usage:

- Use in Candle magic, Herbal bags, Incense, and Spells.
- Invokes spirits.
- Keeps away demons and nightmares while sleeping.
- Protects against wild animals.
- Use in protection and exorcism spells.
- Use on tools to aid divination.

Medicinal attributes: Anti-asthmatic, Antibiotic, Anti-diarrhoea, Antitussive, Bronchodilator, Decongestant, Expectorant.

. . .

Medicinal usage:

- Helps ease asthma, bronchitis, colds, coughs, and whooping cough.
- Relieves congestion from nose, throat, and chest.
- Relieves diarrhoea and soothes haemorrhoids.
- Use the root as a decoction for the treatment of bladder incontinence.
- Works well on respiratory complaints.

80

Nettle

Magical attributes: Curse-breaking, Exorcism, Healing, Protection, Purification.

Magical usage:

- Use in Candle magic, Herbal bags, Incense, and Spells.
- Add to healing and protection charms.
- Burn to remove a curse.
- Carry to remove a curse and send it back.
- Drink the juice or a tea from nettle for purification.
- Sprinkle around the house to keep out evil.
- Use in purification baths.

Medicinal attributes: Anti-diarrhoea, Astringent, Diuretic, Galactagogue, Tonic.

. . .

Medicinal usage:

- A decoction of the plant eases diarrhoea.
- An infusion stimulates the digestive system.
- Apply a decoction of the root to your hair to prevent hair loss.
- Drink to promote milk flow in nursing mothers.
- Helps treat issues with the urinary tract

Warning - Old plants, if used uncooked, can cause kidney damage and the symptoms of poisoning.

81

Nutmeg

Magical attributes: Health, Luck, Money, Prosperity.

Magical usage:

- Use in Candle magic, Herbal bags, Incense, and Spells.
- Carry for good luck.
- Use in money and prosperity spells.

Medicinal attributes: Abortifacient, Analgesic, Anti-diarrhoea, Anti-nausea, Anti-rheumatic, Astringent, Bitter-tonic.

Medicinal usage:

- Apply topically to numb pain.
- Apply to tooth and gums to treat toothache.
- Bathe in or apply as an extract to relieve eczema and rheumatism.
- Can be used to stimulate menstrual flow.
- Relieves catarrh.
- Use to relieve bloating, colic, diarrhoea, gastroenteritis, indigestion, and vomiting.

Warning - Do not use if pregnant.

82

Orris Root

Magical attributes: Divination, Love, Protection, Repels evil spirits.

Magical usage:

- Use in Candle magic, Herbal bags, Incense, and Spells.
- Bathe in roots and leaves for personal protection.
- Hang roots and leaves in the house for protection.
- Offers protection from evil spirits.
- Sprinkle around the house to attract love.
- Use to find love.

Medicinal attributes: Anti-diarrhoea, Antitussive, Bronchodilator, Cathartic, Diaphoretic, Diuretic, Emetic.

• • •

Medicinal usage:

- Apply extract to reduce bruises.
- Drink the tea to treat bronchitis, colds, coughs, and diarrhoea.
- Use as a gargle for sore throats.
- Use in a wash to rejuvenate skin and reduce fine lines and wrinkles.
- Use to fight bad breath.

83

Papaya (Pawpaw)

Magical attributes: Curse-breaking, Healing, Hex-breaking, Increases magical powers, Jinx-breaking, Repels evil spirits.

Magical usage:

- Use in Candle magic, Herbal bags, Incense, and Spells.
- Burn or bathe in a mixture of the leaves with mandrake for a powerful curse, hex, or jinx breaker.
- Place twigs over a door to keep evil out.

Medicinal attributes: Abortifacient, Anti-arthritic, Aphrodisiac Bitter-tonic, Vulnerary.

Medicinal usage:

- Aids with digestive issues.
- Apply to warts, corns, eczema, and hardness of the skin.
- Relieves arthritic pain.
- Use leaves as a poultice on ulcered skin and wounds.

Warning - do not use if pregnant.

84

Parsley

Magical attributes: Fertility, Healing, Lust, Protection, Purification.

Magical usage:

- Use in Candle magic, Herbal bags, Incense, and Spells.
- Eat to promote fertility.
- Sprinkle or place by the door to protect the home.
- Use in a bath for purification.
- Use in healing spells.

Medicinal attributes: Anti-asthmatic, Antispasmodic, Bronchodilator, Carminative, Digestive, Diuretic, Emmenagogue, Expectorant.

. . .

Medicinal usage:

- A tea of parsley can help ease a difficult menstruation.
- Aids with digestion.
- Chew a parsley leaf to fight bad breath.
- Drink as a tea to ease asthma, bronchitis, and coughs.
- Use to bathe conjunctivitis and inflammation around the eyes.

Warning - Do not use if you have kidney problems.

85

Passion Flower

Magical attributes: Emotional balance, Friendship, Love, Peace, Prosperity.

Magical usage:

- Use in Candle magic, Herbal bags, Incense, and Spells.
- Carry to attract friends.
- Place in the house to bring peace and calm arguments.
- Promotes emotional balance and peace.

Medicinal attributes: Anti-arthritic, Anti-inflammatory, Anti-rheumatic, Antiseptic, Carminative, Relaxant, Sedative, Soporific.

· · ·

Medicinal usage:

- Apply to eczema and rashes.
- Drink before bed or apply as an extract to promote restful sleep.
- Eases the pain of arthritis, fibromyalgia, and rheumatism.
- Use as a wash to cleanse skin and ease sunburn.
- Use to bath infected skin.
- Use to calm anxiety and soothe nerves.
- Use to reduce the pain caused by inflammation and muscle strain.

86

Pau D'Arco

Magical attributes: Healing.

Magical usage:

- Use in Candle magic, Herbal bags, Incense, and Spells.
- Add power to the herb by allowing it to absorb moonlight.
- Use in healing rituals, particularly effective for severe illnesses.

Medicinal attributes: Analgesic, Anti-arthritic, Anti-asthmatic, Antibiotic, Anti-inflammatory, Anti-rheumatic, Antiviral, Bronchodilator, Diuretic, Immunostimulant, Sedative, Vulnerary.

. . .

Medicinal usage:

- Boosts the immune system.
- Purifies the blood.
- Relieves arthritis, asthma, bronchitis, gastritis, periodontitis, and rheumatism.
- Strong antibiotic and antiviral.
- Use as a gargle for mouth ulcers, periodontitis, and sore throats.
- Use bark as a poultice and apply to eczema, haemorrhoids, infections, psoriasis, skin inflammations, and wounds.

87

Pennyroyal

Magical attributes: Astral Projection, Money, Peace, Protection, Travel safety.

Magical usage:

- Use in Candle magic, Herbal bags, Incense, and Spells.
- Burn for protection during astral travel, meditation, spells, and rituals.
- Carry to attract money and bring about positive results in business.
- Carry to ease seasickness.
- Carry to repel negative energy.

Medicinal attributes: Abortifacient, Antitussive, Bitter-tonic, Expectorant, Decongestant.

. . .

Medicinal usage:

- Apply as an extract to tighten skin.
- Eases coughs and congestion.
- Relieves headaches.
- Relieves indigestion and stomach cramps.
- Stimulates menstruation when consumed.
- Trusted cold remedy.
- Use as a gargle for periodontitis.

Warning - Do not use if pregnant.

88

Peppermint

Magical attributes: Healing, Love, Prophetic dreams, Psychic abilities, Purification, Sleep.

Magical usage:

- Use in Candle magic, Herbal bags, Incense, and Spells.
- Place under your pillow for prophetic dreams.
- Use in healing and purification baths.

Medicinal attributes: Anaesthetic, Anti-asthmatic, Anti-nausea, Anti-rheumatic, Antiseptic, Bitter-tonic, Bronchodilator, decongestant, Depurative, Diaphoretic, Digestive, Refrigerant.

Medicinal usage:

- Apply as a rub to ease pancreatitis.
- Apply as a cream or poultice to relieve and soothe burns, itching skin, neuralgia, and rheumatism.
- Apply as an extract or rub to ease bronchitis, sinusitis, and upper respiratory tract infections.
- Drink as a tea to help relieve morning sickness.
- Eases heartburn, an upset stomach, and nausea.
- Ingesting helps with digestive issues including cramping, colic, dyspepsia, flatulence, gastritis, irritable bowel syndrome, and stomach ulcers.
- Purifies the blood.
- Relieves motion sickness.
- Relieves symptoms during colds and flu.
- Use as a gargle to fight bad breath.

89

Pine

Magical attributes: Healing, Fertility, Money, Prosperity, Repels negative energy, Strength, Wisdom.

Magical usage:

- Use in Candle magic, Herbal bags, Incense, and Spells.
- Burn for strength and to remove negative energies.
- Draws steady money.
- Removes negative mental energy.
- Spiritual cleanser.

Medicinal attributes: Analgesic, Anti-rheumatic, Antiseptic, Antitussive, Bronchodilator, Diuretic, Expectorant.

Medicinal usage:

- Apply as an extract to muscular pain including rheumatism.
- Apply topically to improve blood flow to the area of application.
- Drink or eat to ease respiratory problems.
- Effective against bronchitis, coughs and colds.

90

Ragwort (Tansy)

Magical attributes: Protection, Repels evil spirits.

Magical usage:

- Use in Candle magic, Herbal bags, Incense, and Spells.
- Burn to repel evil spirits.
- Carry for protection.

Medicinal attributes: Abortifacient, Anti-arthritic, Anti-inflammatory, Anti-rheumatic, Emmenagogue.

Medicinal usage:

- Apply as a poultice or rub to relieve backache.

- Apply as a rub to areas of inflammation.
- Apply as an extract to reduce blemishes and bruises.
- Apply topically to treat fibromyalgia.
- Encourages menstruation.
- Use as a compress for arthritis and rheumatism.

Warning - Can be fatal if ingested, only use under medical supervision.

Warning - Do not use if pregnant.

91

Raspberry Leaf

Magical attributes: Healing, Love, Protection, Sleep, Visions

Magical usage:

- Use in Candle magic, Herbal bags, Incense, and Spells.
- Burn to aid with visions.
- Carry for healing.
- Place under the pillow to aid with sleep.

Medicinal attributes: Abortifacient, Anti-diarrhoea, Anti-nausea, Childbirth, Galactagogue, Tonic.

Medicinal usage:

- Apply as a compress or wash to ease eczema, rashes, and sunburn.
- Eases menstrual problems.
- Eases nausea and vomiting.
- Helps milk flow in nursing mothers.
- Use from week 32 of pregnancy to ease childbirth and labour.

Warning - Do until final trimester of pregnancy, midwife recommendations state it is safe to use after 32 weeks.

92

Red Clover

Magical attributes: Beauty, Clairvoyance, Exorcism, Fidelity, Love, Luck, Money, Protection, Repels negative energy, Success.

Magical usage:

- Use in Candle magic, Herbal bags, Incense, and Spells.
- Carry to attract love and money.
- Improves clairvoyance abilities.
- Sprinkle around the house to banish evil spirits and negative energy.
- Use for rituals to enhance beauty and youth.

Medicinal attributes: Anti-arthritic, Antibacterial, Anti-inflammatory, Antitussive, Bronchodilator, Depurative, Expectorant, Immunostimulant, Vulnerary.

. . .

Medicinal usage:

- Boosts the immune system.
- Eases arthritis.
- Eases bronchitis, coughs, and whooping cough.
- Fights off bacterial infections.
- Purifies the blood.
- Reduces hot flushes caused by menopause.
- Relieves the pain of burns, eczema, psoriasis, and sores.

93

Rosary Pea (Crab's Eye)

Magical attributes: Luck, Protection, Repels the evil eye.

Magical usage:

- Use in Candle magic, Herbal bags, Incense, and Spells.
- Carry or place in amulets for good luck.
- Wear to protect against the evil eye.

Medicinal usage: Abortifacient, Analgesic, Antipyretic, Antitussive, Aphrodisiac, Astringent, Diuretic, Emetic, Expectorant, Laxative, Purgative, Refrigerant, Sedative.

Medicinal attributes:

- A tea from the leaves eases colds, coughs, and fevers.
- A tea from the roots treats gonorrhoea and jaundice.
- Apply the seeds as a poultice to ease paralysis, sciatica, and stiff joints.
- Use the extract from the seed to promote hair growth.

Warning - Do not use if pregnant.

Warning - Seeds are poisonous do not consume.

94

Rose Hips (Dog Rose)

Magical attributes: Balance, Divination, Healing, Love, Luck, Peace, Protection, Psychic abilities, Purification.

Magical usage:

- Use in Candle magic, Herbal bags, Incense, and Spells.
- Add to healing spells and bags to boost healing.
- Place around the house to balance energies and bring peace.
- Use in a cleansing, purifying bath.
- Wear to attract love.

Medicinal attributes: Anti-arthritic, Anti-diarrhoea, Anti-inflammatory, Anti-rheumatic, Antitussive, Astringent, Carminative, Decongestant, Diuretic, Laxative, Tonic.

· · ·

Medicinal usage:

- Apply topically to reduce fine lines and wrinkles.
- Apply topically to reduce scars.
- Eases colds, congestion, coughs, and flu.
- Eases menstrual problems.
- Helps relieve diarrhoea and urinary tract problems.
- Treats arthritis and rheumatism.
- Wash in an infusion to re-hydrate the skin.

95

Rose Petals

Magical attributes: Healing, Love, Luck, Peace, Prophetic dreams, Protection, Psychic abilities, Youth.

Magical usage:

- Use in Candle magic, Herbal bags, Incense, and Spells.
- Drink rose tea before bed to encourage prophetic dreams.
- Place around the house for domestic peace.
- Use in a bath to attract love.
- Use in love spells of all kinds.
- Use in a wash or bath to stay young.

Medicinal attributes: Anti-asthmatic, Anti-diarrhoea, Antitussive, Bitter-tonic, Bronchodilator, Diaphoretic, Diuretic, Emollient, Sedative, Soporific, Vulnerary.

. . .

Medicinal usage:

- Apply as a poultice to abrasions, sores, and wounds.
- Drink as a tea to treat asthma, bronchitis, coughs, and fever.
- Drink before bed to combat insomnia.
- Helps relieve dizziness, headaches, and menstrual cramps.
- Take to ease diarrhoea, dysmenorrhoea, indigestion, and urinary tract infections.
- Use as a gargle to treat mouth sores.
- Uses as a wash or extract on dermatitis, eczema, and rashes.

96

Rosemary

Magical attributes: Exorcism, Healing, Love, Lust, Protection, Purification, Sleep, Youth.

Magical usage:

- Use in Candle magic, Herbal bags, Incense, and Spells.
- Burn to cleanse and purify an area.
- Use for all kinds of healing.
- Use in a bath to attract love and keep you young.
- Use in love and lust incenses and potions.

Medicinal attributes: Analgesic, Antibacterial, Antidepressant, Antifungal, Anti-inflammatory, Antioxidant, Anti-rheumatic, Antispasmodic, Antiviral, Depurative, Digestive, Rubefacient, Stimulant.

. . .

Medicinal usage:

- Aids circulation.
- Aids digestion.
- Apply to fine lines and wrinkles.
- Apply topically for increase blood flow to that area.
- Eases flatulence.
- Improves brain function.
- Purifies the blood.
- Relieves depression and headaches.
- Relieves rheumatism.
- Use as a gargle to treat bad breath.

97

Rowan

Magical attributes: Increases magical powers, Protection, Psychic abilities, Luck.

Magical usage:

- Use in Candle magic, Herbal bags, Incense, and Spells.
- Make ritual tools using rowan to increase their power.
- Carry for protection.

Medicinal attributes: Anti-diarrhoea, Bitter-tonic, Bronchodilator, Diuretic.

Medicinal usage:

- Helps to relieve cold and flu.
- Helps to relieve diarrhoea.
- Relieves digestive issues.

Note - large quantities can be poisonous. Always use as a decoction.

98

Saffron

Magical attributes: Healing, Love, Wind spells.

Magical usage:

- Use in Candle magic, Herbal bags, Incense, and Spells.
- Keep in the home to bring happiness.
- Wear or carry for healing.

Medicinal attributes: Abortifacient, Analgesic, Anti-asthmatic, Antidepressant, Anti-rheumatic, Antispasmodic, Antitussive, Aphrodisiac, Bitter-tonic, Carminative, Diaphoretic, Emmenagogue, Expectorant, Carminative Sedative, Soporific, Stimulant.

Medicinal usage:

- Apply to haemorrhoids, sores, and snakebites.
- Drink as a tea to ease headaches.
- Drink before bed to combat insomnia.
- Eases colic and flatulence.
- Eases menstruation.
- Fights depression.
- Helps ease the pain of neuralgia and rheumatism
- Relieves asthma, cough, and fever.
- Use as a wash to lighten the complexion.

Warning - Do not use if pregnant.

99

Sage

Magical attributes: Healing, Immortality, Longevity, Money, Prosperity, Protection, Purification, Repels negative energy, Wisdom.

Magical usage:

- Use in Candle magic, Herbal bags, Incense, and Spells.
- Burn to purify and cleanse an area and repel negative energies.
- Use in money spells.
- Use in healing spells.
- Use to cleanse a home.

Medicinal attributes: Anti-inflammatory, Antioxidant, Antiseptic, Antitussive, Bitter, Bitter-tonic, Digestive, Relaxant, Vulnerary.

. . .

Medicinal usage:

- Aids digestion.
- Dries up milk in mothers no longer wishing to nurse.
- Eases and helps to regulate menstruation.
- Eases muscle and joint pain.
- Heals wounds.
- Improves brain function.
- Relieves allergies.
- Relieves colds and fever.
- Slows down the aging process.
- Use as a gargle to relieve a sore throat and treat mouth infections.
- Use to darken hair colour.
- Use to wash cuts and sores.

100

Scotch Broom Leaf

Magical attributes: Exorcism, Protection, Psychic abilities, Purification, Wind spells.

Magical usage:

- Use in Candle magic, Herbal bags, Incense, and Spells.
- Burn to calm the wind.
- Drink as a tea to improve psychic abilities.
- Sprinkle to banish evil spirits.
- Use in purification and protection spells
- Use the branches to make a traditional besom.

Medicinal attributes: Abortifacient, Analgesic, Anti-inflammatory, Diuretic.

. . .

Medicinal usage:

- Apply topically to ease joint pain.
- Apply extract to tooth and gums to relieve toothache.
- Helps treat fevers, gout, and malaria.

Warning - Do not use if pregnant

Warning - Toxic in large doses

101

Shavegrass (Horsetail)

Magical attributes: Fertility.

Magical usage:

- Use in Candle magic, Herbal bags, Incense, and Spells.
- Keep some in the bedroom or place under the bed when trying to conceive.
- Use in fertility spells.

Medicinal attributes: Anti-inflammatory, Antioxidant, Astringent, Bitter-tonic, Demulcent, Diuretic, Immunostimulant.

Medicinal usage:

- Apply topically to acne, athlete's foot, boils, burns, chilblains, frostbite, rashes, and ulcers.
- Boosts the immune system.
- Can be used to treat malaria.
- Drink as a treat to help with urinary tract infections.
- Eases bronchitis, fever, and respiratory infections.
- Helps strengthen bones, hair, and nails.
- Helps to quicken the healing of broken bones.
- Reduces fevers.
- Use as a wash on swollen eyes.
- Use in a wash to reduce oily skin.
- Use to treat bladder problems, dyspepsia, and kidney stones.
- Used to control bleeding, internally and externally.

102

Spanish Moss (Grandfather's whiskers)

Magical attributes: Exorcism, Luck, Money, Visions.

Magical usage:

- Use in Candle magic, Herbal bags, Incense, and Spells.
- Carry for good luck.
- Place around home or burn to banish poltergeists.
- Drink as an extract to assist with visions.

Medicinal attributes:

Medicinal usage: Analgesic, Antipyretic.

- Drink as a tea to treat chills and fevers.
- Eases contraction pains during birth.
- Wash in an infusion to rejuvenate skin and combat fine lines and wrinkles.

103

St. John's Wort

Magical attributes: Courage, Divination, Exorcism, Happiness, Health, Love, Protection, Strength.

Magical usage:

- Use in Candle magic, Herbal bags, Incense, and Spells.
- Carry for courage.
- Use in protection and exorcism spells.
- Use the leaves in a necklace to ward off ill health.

Medicinal attributes: Anaesthetic, Analgesic, Antidepressant, Anti-inflammatory, Antiseptic, Astringent, Carminative, Sedative, Soporific, Vulnerary.

Medicinal usage:

- Apply to areas suffering from nerve damage, bruises, burns, sprains, sores, and wounds.
- Drink and apply to ease cold sores, herpes and shingles.
- Drink as a tea for nerve pain, sciatica, and stomach problems.
- Drink before bed to help with insomnia.
- Eases anxiety and nerves.
- Relieves tension headaches.
- Relieves the symptoms of Crohn's disease and irritable bowel syndrome.
- Use as a tea to treat depression.

104

Star Anise

Magical attributes: Luck, Protection, Psychic abilities, Purification, Repels the evil eye, Youth.

Magical usage:

- Use in Candle magic, Herbal bags, Incense, and Spells.
- Burn or wear seeds to increase psychic abilities.
- Place in good luck charms.
- Place inside pillow to keep away nightmares.
- Use in purification baths.
- Wards off the evil eye.

Medicinal attributes: Antispasmodic, Antitussive, Bitter-tonic, Bronchodilator, Expectorant, Galactagogue, Stimulant.

. . .

Medicinal usage:

- Aids with menopausal problems.
- Cooled tea can be sponged on the face to lighten the complexion.
- Fights bad breath.
- Increases milk production for nursing women.
- Relieves flatulence.
- Treats bronchitis, colds, coughs, flu, and sinusitis.
- Use topically as an antiseptic.
- Use with eucalyptus as a chest rub for bronchitis and respiratory problems.
- Use with peppermint to treat colic.

105

Sweet Cicely (Shepherd's needle)

Magical attributes: Happiness, Purification.

Magical usage:

- Use in Candle magic, Herbal bags, Incense, and Spells.
- Use for cleansing ritual tools.
- Drink to promote happiness.
- Scatter with cremated ashes, or on a grave to bring peace to the dead.
- Protects against elf-shot

Medicinal attributes: Abortifacient, Antiseptic, Antispasmodic,

Antitussive, Bitter-tonic, Carminative, Decongestant, Expectorant, Galactagogue Soporific, Vulnerary.

. . .

Medicinal usage:

- Apply the roots as a poultice to infected wounds.
- Can cause onset of menstruation.
- Drink the extract with warm milk before bed to promote sleep and ease insomnia.
- Drink to relieve colic, flatulence, indigestion.
- Eases and helps prevent 'elf-shot', a sudden unexplained shooting pain in the body.
- Eases coughs.
- Increases milk production in nursing mothers.
- Relieves cramps and spasms.
- Relieves congestion in nose throat and chest.
- The leaves are sweet and can be eaten to satisfy sugar cravings.
- Use the roots to treat gout.

Warning - Do not use if pregnant.

106

Tea

Magical attributes: Divination, Courage, Prosperity, Strength.

Magical usage:

- Use in Candle magic, Herbal bags, Incense, and Spells.
- The leaves can be used for divination.
- Use the leaves in money spells.

Medicinal attributes: Anti-asthmatic, Anti-diarrhoea, Antioxidant, Expectorant, Decongestant, Sedative.

Medicinal usage:

- Eases asthma.
- Has a calming effect on the body.
- Relieves colds and congestion.
- Relieves diarrhoea, tooth decay, and help prevents tissue damage from radiation therapy.

107

Thistle (Scotch Thistle)

Magical attributes: Anti-hex, Energy, Healing, Hex-breaking,

Money, Protection, Joy.

Magical usage:

- Use in Candle magic, Herbal bags, Incense, and Spells.
- Burn extract from the seeds during protection spells.
- Burn the flowers for protection.
- Burn to break and counteract hexes.
- Carry the flowers for energy, joy, and protection.
- Hang in the home to keep away unwanted visitors.
- Use in Protection spells, also used to bring spiritual and financial blessings.

Medicinal attributes: Astringent, Carminative.

Medicinal usage:

- Apply the juice to treat ulcers.
- Drink a tea from the leaves and roots to ease anxiety and nerves.
- Use a decoction made from the root to help stop bleeding.
- Use the leaves and roots to treat rickets.

108

Thyme

Magical attributes: Healing, Health, Purification, Psychic abilities, Repels negative energy.

Magical usage:

- Use in Candle magic, Herbal bags, Incense, and Spells.
- Burn as purification incense.
- Burn to promote good health.
- Hang in the home to banish negative energies and for purification.
- Use in healing spells.
- Wear to increase Psychic abilities.

Medicinal attributes: Antibacterial, Antifungal, Antiseptic, Antitussive, Anti-viral, Bitter-tonic, Decongestant, Digestive, Expectorant, Vulnerary.

. . .

Medicinal usage:

- Apply fresh leaves to cuts and wounds.
- Apply to bruises.
- Drink an infusion made from the leaves to aid digestion and relieve flatulence, dyspepsia, and indigestion.
- Eases coughs, emphysema, and whooping cough.
- Eases cramps.
- Eases menstrual cramps.
- Relieves congestion in nose, throat, and chest.
- Relieves symptoms of cold and flu.
- Use as a gargle for bad breath, tonsillitis, and sore throat.

109

Valerian Root (All-heal)

Magical attributes: Anti-curse, Anti-hex, Dream magic, Harmony, Healing, Protection, Purification.

Magical usage:

- Use in Candle magic, Herbal bags, Incense, and Spells.
- Adds power to curses or hexes.
- Drink as a tea to balance energy and purify yourself.
- Keep in the home to bring harmony.
- Sprinkle at front door and say their name to keep away unwanted visitors.
- Use as protection against curses and hexes.
- Use in love spells.
- Use in purification baths.
- Use in healing spells.

Medicinal   attributes: Analgesic,   Anti-rheumatic,
Antispasmodic,   Bitter-tonic,   Decongestant,   Expectorant,
Carminative, Relaxant, Sedative, Vulnerary.

Medicinal usage:

- Aids a restful sleep.
- Apply to acne, bruises, and wounds.
- Eases congestion in the nose, throat, and chest.
- Eases migraines.
- Relieves colic and flatulence.
- Relieves rheumatism.
- Treats colds.
- Use in a bath to ease muscle cramps and spasms.
- Use to treat nervous conditions including hysteria,
  post-traumatic stress, and shock.

110

Vanilla

Magical attributes: Energy, Lust, Love, Mental focus.

Magical usage:

- Use in Candle magic, Herbal bags, Incense, and Spells.
- Carry to increase energy and mental focus.
- Use in love charms and spells.
- Wear to attract love.

Medicinal attributes: Anaesthetic, Antibacterial, Antifungal, Anti-inflammatory, Antioxidant, Aphrodisiac, Vulnerary

Medicinal usage:

- Apply to acne and spots.
- Apply to burns, cuts, and wounds.
- Apply to tooth and gums to reduce toothache.
- Use in a wash to slow signs of aging and reduce fine lines and wrinkles.

111

Verbena Leaf (Lemon Verbena)

Magical attributes: Love, Protection, Purification, Strength.

Magical usage:

- Use in Candle magic, Herbal bags, Incense, and Spells.
- Add to increase power of any magical working.
- Use Elecampane, Mistletoe, and Verbena to create a medieval true love powder.
- Use in a purification and protection bath.
- Wear to attract love.

Medicinal attributes: Anti-asthmatic, Anti-diarrhoea, Antipyretic, Bitter-tonic, Carminative, Sedative, Soporific.

. . .

Medicinal usage:

- Apply as an extract or poultice on varicose veins.
- Drink as a tea to reduce fevers
- Drink as a tea to relieve colic, flatulence, and indigestion.
- Drink before bed to relieve insomnia.
- Soothes Anxiety and nerves
- Use as a wash for skin conditions including acne, eczema, and spots.

112

Vervain (Blue Vervain)

Magical attributes: Healing, Protection, Prosperity, Purification.

Magical usage:

- Use in Candle magic, Herbal bags, Incense, and Spells.
- Carry for protection.
- Place under the pillow to repel nightmares.
- Use in all kinds of protection spells.
- Use in purification baths.

Medicinal attributes: Abortifacient, Analgesic, Anti-asthmatic, Astringent, Antispasmodic, Bronchodilator, Decongestant, Depurative, Diuretic, Emmenagogue, Expectorant, Galactagogue, Carminative, Sedative, Vulnerary.

. . .

Medicinal usage:

- Apply to eczema, insect bites, rashes, sores, and wounds.
- Can encourage menstruation.
- Eases congestion in nose, throat, and chest.
- Eases earache, headaches, and migraines.
- Eases menstruation.
- Increases milk production in nursing mothers.
- Purifies the blood.
- Relieves anxiety and nerves.
- Relieves asthma, bronchitis, and pneumonia.
- Relieves symptoms of cold and flu.
- Use as a rinse or gargle for bleeding gums, gingivitis, mouth ulcers, and sore throat.

Warning - Do not use if pregnant.

113

White Clover

Magical attributes: Curse-breaking, Purification.

Magical usage:

- Use in Candle magic, Herbal bags, Incense, and Spells.
- Put in each corner of a room when breaking curses or reversing spells.
- Wear to break curses.

Medicinal attributes:, Anti-arthritic, Antitussive, Anti-inflammatory, Bronchodilator, Depurative, Vulnerary.

Medicinal usage:

- Apply as a poultice or extract to ease arthritis, gout, inflammation, and psoriasis
- Apply to sores and wounds.
- Drink as a tea for arthritis, coughs, colds, gout, and fevers.
- Helps to relieve bronchitis, coughs, and whooping cough.
- Purifies the blood.

114

White Willow Bark

Magical attributes: Divination, Healing, Love, Protection.

Magical usage:

- Use in Candle magic, Herbal bags, Incense, and Spells.
- Carry and use in spells to attract love.
- To intensify its power, leave in the moonlight for three nights.
- Use the leaves, bark, and wood in healing spells.

Medicinal attributes: Analgesic, Anti-arthritic, Anti-diarrhoea, Anti-inflammatory, Anti-rheumatic, Antiseptic, Astringent, Diaphoretic, Relaxant, Vulnerary.

Medicinal usage:

- A remedy for bladder problems, diarrhoea, kidney irritations, and urinary tract infections.
- Apply to burns, cuts, sores, and wounds.
- Eases gout and neuralgia.
- Eases muscle and joint pain.
- Helps relieve menstrual cramps and toothache.
- Reduces arthritis and rheumatic inflammation.
- Reduces fevers.
- Relieves acute and chronic pain.
- Relieves backache, headaches, migraines, and neck pain.
- Use as a gargle for sore gums, sore throat, and tonsillitis.

Warning - Do not use if taking aspirin

Warning - Pregnant and nursing women should not use without first seeking medical opinion.

115

Wolfsbane

Magical attributes: Protection.

Magical usage:

- Use in Candle magic, Herbal bags, Incense, and Spells.
- Used in sympathetic magic.
- Used to protect the home from werewolves and prevent shapeshifting.

Medicinal attributes:

Medicinal usage:

. . .

Warning - Highly poisonous. Even small amounts taken orally or absorbed through skin can kill. If you must use this herb always use gloves.

116

Yarrow Flower

Magical attributes: Courage, Divination, Healing, Love, Repels negative energy.

Magical usage:

- Use in Candle magic, Herbal bags, Incense, and Spells.
- Aids in divination.
- Carried to repel negative energy and influences.
- Place in a red cloth with a written note of your fears to grant you the courage to face them.
- Use in love charms.

Medicinal attributes: Antibacterial, Antibiotic, Anti-diarrhoea, Anti-inflammatory, Antiseptic, Astringent, Antitussive, Depurative, Diaphoretic, Digestive, Diuretic, Vulnerary.

. . .

Medicinal usage:

- Aids digestion.
- Apply to cleaned burns, cuts, ulcers, and wounds.
- Apply to infected wounds to fight the infection and promote healing.
- Apply topically to reduce varicose veins and haemorrhoids
- Good remedy for colds.
- Helps to relieve cystitis and irritable bladder.
- Purifies the blood.
- Relieves coughs, colds, fever, and flu.
- Relieves diarrhoea.
- Soothes painful joints.
- Use as a wash to clear the skin.
- Use on athlete's foot.
- Use with shampoo to prevent baldness.

Healing and Magical
Properties of Colours

117

Colours in Healing and Magic

Light is just one small part of the energy around us, and colour is simply the wavelength and frequencies of the electromagnetic spectrum of light that we can see.

Colour healing works on the principal that each colour possesses its own unique wavelength. Simply looking at a colour causes changes in the body due to how the eyes transmit the data to the brain. Each wavelength has its own frequency and thus is processed differently and brings about different changes. But the application of colour therapy doesn't just stop with visual stimulation. Colours can be placed on specific areas, where the body reacts to the energy created by their wavelengths.

Colours have been used for healing since at least the time of ancient Egypt and Greece. There have been documents found dating back to approximately 1550BC detailing the use of colours in healing treatments. However, over exposure to a colour can also bring about negative changes, so care must be taken.

A good example to use of the proven benefits of electromagnetic energy are gamma rays, these are another part of the electromagnetic spectrum with a shorter wavelength than visible light. Gamma rays are not only used to kill cancer cells but also to sterilise medical equipment.

Colours have also been used in magical practices to draw specific energies and intentions to create a desired result. Such practices range from altar dressings and candle magic, to herbal bags. Choosing the right colour for your desire can be as important as the working itself and aid in the gathering of appropriate energies and intentions.

The following section has a list of the main colours and details their usage broken down into the following categories.

Positive aspects - shows the mental and magical changes exposure can create

Negative aspects - shows the negative mental changes over-exposure can create

Works well on - details the best medicinal applications for the colour.

Black

Positive Aspects: Banishing negativity, Curse-breaking, Divination, Efficiency, Emotional safety, Glamour, Grounding, Hex-breaking, Learning, Protection, Repelling black magic, Safety, Security, Spell-breaking, Spell reversing, Wisdom.

Negative Aspects: Coldness, Heaviness, Menace, Oppression.

Chakra: Root.

Chakra Element: Earth.

Magical Element: Spirit.

Works well on: Foot problems, Pain relief.

Blue

Positive Aspects: Astral projection, Calmness, Communication, Efficiency, Fidelity, Mental focus, Intelligence, Logic, Protection, Reflection, Removing negative energy, Serenity, Sincerity, Trust, Truth, Weight loss, Willpower.

Negative Aspects: Coldness, Lack of emotion, Unfriendliness.

Chakra: Throat.

Chakra Element: Ether.

Magical Element: Water.

Works well on: Arms, Bleeding, Fevers, Hands, Hyperactivity, Inflammation, Neck, Pain, Throat.

Brown

Positive Aspects: House blessing, Animal magic, Earth magic, Concentration, Patience, Stability, Stamina, Grounding.

Negative Aspects: Arrogance, Complacency, Inflexibility, Lack of diversity, Lack of spontaneity.

Chakra: Root

Chakra Element: Earth

Magical Element: Earth

Works well on: Hyperactivity, and helps to stabilise the system.

Gold

Positive Aspects: Abundance, Attraction, Divination, Fortune, Health, Justice, Luxury, Male energy, Masculine divinity, Positive attitude, Prosperity, Solar energy, Understanding.

Negative Aspects: Addiction, Aggression, Domineering, Greed.

Chakra: Solar Plexus.

Chakra Element: Fire.

Magical Element: Fire.

Works well on: Boosts immune system, Cardiac problems, Curing additions, Endocrine system, Strengthens other colours.

Green

Positive Aspects: Abundance, Acceptance, Balance, Emotional healing, Growth, Harmony, Luck, Marriage, Money, Peace, Physical healing, Prosperity, Reassurance, Refreshment, Restoration.

Negative Aspects: Boredom, Stagnation.

Chakra: Heart.

Chakra Element: Air.

Magical Element: Earth.

Works well on: Breathing problems, Burn pains, Chest, Circulation, Congestion, Germs, Headaches, Heart, Lungs, Neuralgia, Pituitary gland, Skin conditions, Touch sensitivity, Ulcers, Wound healing.

Grey

Positive Aspects: Psychological neutrality contemplation, Removing negative influence

Negative Aspects: Depression, Lack of energy, Lack of confidence,

Chakra: N/A.

Chakra Element: N/A.

Magical Element: Water

Works well on: Although grey has no healing benefits it can be used to reduce the impact of other colours.

Indigo

Positive Aspects: Ambition, Clarity, Connection to higher self, Dignity, Divination, Insight, Meditation, Psychic abilities, Spiritual guidance, Spirituality.

Negative Aspects: Fearful, Intolerance, Isolation, Judgmental.

Chakra: Third eye.

Chakra Element: Light.

Magical Element: Water.

Works well on: Boosting the immune system, Haemorrhoids, Pain relief, Pituitary gland, Thyroid problems, Varicose veins,

Orange

Positive Aspects: Abundance, Fun, Creativity, Intellectual matters, Joy, Opportunity, Passion, Physical comfort, Security, self-expression, Sensuality, Vitality, Warmth.

Negative Aspects: Deprivation, Frustration, Immaturity.

Chakra: Sacral.

Chakra Element: Water.

Magical Element: Fire.

Works well on: Appetite, Digestive disorders, Kidneys, Liver, Lumbar Plexus, Pancreas, Relieving flatulence, Bladder, Relieving spasms and cramps, Reproductive system, Respiratory problems, Sexual organs, Stimulating stomach, Thyroid problems, Weight issues.

Pink

Positive Aspects: Compassion, Domestic harmony, Emotional healing, Femininity, Friendship, Love, Maturity, Nurture, Partnership, Physical tranquillity, Protection of children, Romance, Self-improvement, Sexuality, Spiritual healing, Warmth.

Negative Aspects: Emasculation, Emotional claustrophobia, Inhibition, Physical weakness.

Chakra: Heart.

Chakra Element: Air.

Magical Element: Fire.

Works well on: Bones, General health, Grief, Joints, Kidneys, Physical heart issues, Sadness, Uterus.

Purple

Positive Aspects: Drive away evil, Independence, Influence, Psychic abilities, Sensitivity, Spiritual power, Wisdom.

Negative Aspects: Delusions of grandeur, Depression, Irritability.

Chakra: Crown.

Chakra Element: Spirit.

Magical Element: Water.

Works well on: Anxiety, Exhaustion, Headaches, Low self-esteem, Migraines, Obsessions, Stress.

Red:

Positive Aspects: Assertiveness, Courage, Energy, Fertility, Independence, Passion, Stimulating, Strength, Survival, Warmth.

Negative Aspects: Aggression.

Chakra: Root.

Chakra Element: Earth.

Magical Element: Fire.

Works well on: Anaemia, Ankles, Bladder, Bones, Bowels, Chills, Feet, Legs, Liver problems, Lymph system, Nose, Teeth.

Silver

Positive Aspects: Communication, Dreams, Emotional stability, Female energy, Feminine divinity, Intuition, Meditation, Moon magic, Neutralise negativity, Psychic abilities, Rebirth, Reincarnation, Stability,

Negative Aspects: Indecisive, Insincere, Non-committal.

Chakra: Crown.

Chakra Element: Spirit.

Magical Element: Water

Works well on: Anxiety, Boosts health benefits of other colours, Menstruation problems, Nervous tension.

Violet

Positive Aspects: Authenticity, Containment, Luxury, Quality, Spiritual awareness, Truth, Vision.

Negative Aspects: Decadence, Inferiority, Introversion, Suppression.

Chakra: Crown.

Chakra Element: Spirit.

Magical Element: Spirit.

Works well on: Bladder, Hyperactivity, Insomnia, Isolation, Loneliness, Nervous disorders, Relationships, Spiritual wellbeing, Spleen, Suppressing the appetite, White blood cells.

White

Positive Aspects: All purpose, Balance, Clarity, Cleansing, Healing, Innocence, Peace, Purity, Simplicity, Spirituality, Truth, Unity.

Negative Aspects: Coldness, Sterility, Superiority, Unfriendliness.

Chakra: All Chakras.

Chakra Element: All elements.

Magical Element: Spirit.

Works well on: All-purpose healing, Pain relief, Strengthens colours it is used with.

Yellow

Positive Aspects: Charm, Concentration, Confidence, Creativity. Pleasure, Ego, Emotional strength, Flexibility, Friendliness, Happiness, Imagination, Inspiration, Learning, Memory, Optimism, Persuasion, Self-esteem, Solar magic, Success, Travel safety.

Negative Aspects: Anxiety, Depression, Emotional fragility, Fear, Irrationality.

Chakra: Solar Plexus.

Chakra Element: Fire.

Magical Element: Air.

Works well on: Diabetes, Ears, Eyes, Face, Gall bladder, Heart, Indigestion, Large intestine, Liver, Muscular system, Nerves, Nervous exhaustion, Pancreas, Skin, Solar plexus, Stomach.

Making Magical Items

133

Making a Herbal bag

Herbal bags have been around for as long as there has been belief in magic and the healing powers of Mother Nature. They can be made by anyone and, despite common misconceptions, are not linked to a specific religion or practice. The most important thing whilst making one is the intention.

Once made they can be given to anyone to attract the attributes it was crafted to. It is recommended that they are carried, close to the skin if possible. They can also be placed under your pillow at night.

You will need:

- Coloured cloth.
- Herbs which suit your purpose.
- Needle and thread.
- Paper and pen.
- Ribbon.

Method:

1. First select a coloured piece of cloth which best fits
   your purpose, refer to the 'Healing and Magical
   Properties of Colours' section in this book for
   guidance.
2. Hand sew a small palm sized bag while concentrating
   on your intention. Include either a coloured ribbon
   drawstring at the top or leave a flap so you can sew it
   together once you have finished. If you don't like
   sewing you can always buy a small bag, or even use a
   coloured envelope.
3. Choose the herbs which best suit your purpose.
   Ensure there are no less than three herbs. but no
   more than nine.
4. Place each herb in the bag focusing your intention
   into them as you add them.
5. Place a small piece of paper with the name of the
   person, and the intention of the Herbal bag, inside.
6. Pull the drawstring closed and tie it, or if you opted
   for a flap, sew it together.
7. Visualise a powerful light entering you through the
   crown of your head, passing down to your third eye,
   throat, heart, solar plexus, sacred, and finally your
   root chakra.
8. Visualise this light flowing through your fingers and
   into the contents of the Herbal bag and focus your
   thoughts on the intention.
9. When you feel you are finished, visualise a protective
   light surrounding the bag.
10. Give thanks to the forces you believe in, or simply to
    the energy for helping with your desire.
11. The Herbal bag is now complete and can be given to
    the intended person.

Note: To add additional power to your Herbal bag, use a thread of a different colour, preferably one which boosts the required positive attributes of the intended purpose.

134

Making a Herbal Candle

You will need

- An appropriately coloured candle.
- Dried or fresh herb trimmings.
- Mortar and pestle.
- Vegetable oil.
- Your chosen herbs in extract or tincture form.

Method:

1. Select a coloured candle appropriate to your intention, see the section on 'Healing and Magical Properties of Colours' for guidance.
2. Chop your selected herbs into fine pieces.
3. Use a mortar and pestle to crush and grind the selected herbs as much as possible.
4. Mix 3-6 drops of your herbal extract with the vegetable oil.
5. Anoint the candle with this oil until you have applied it to the whole candle.

6. Now roll the candle in the ground herb mixture so that it sticks onto the candle.
7. The candle is now ready to use.

Never leave a burning candle unattended.

135

Making Incense

You will need:

- Dried or powdered herbs of choice.
- Makko (incense powder).
- Mortar and pestle.
- Water.

Method:

1. Using your mortar and pestle grind your desired herbs into a fine powder. (Alternatively buy powdered versions if available.).
2. Mix with Makko (it should be about 10 - 15 % Makko).
3. Use a sieve to remove any large lumps.
4. Add warm water a few drops at a time and knead using the pestle to form a doughy mixture.
5. Once the texture is smooth shape into cones (if you want a stick you can roll it onto bamboo sticks).
6. Leave to dry for around ten days.

If it doesn't hold together add more Makko.

If it is too dry, add more water.

It is always good practise to keep a list of quantity and weight, that way if your incense doesn't burn well, or burns too fiercely, you can alter the Makko content.

136

Making a Pomander

Pomanders are an aromatic, attractive, old-fashioned gift for protection, strength, and warding off ill health.

You will need:

- An orange.
- Coloured ribbon.
- Cloves.
- Toothpick or tapestry needle. (optional).

Method:

1. Choose a colour of ribbon that best suits your intention, see the 'Healing and Magical Properties of Colours' for guidance.
2. Use the toothpick or needle to poke holes into the orange where you want to add the cloves, you can experiment with different patterns or symbols.

3. Wipe the excess juice off, some people like to roll the orange in cinnamon at this point.

4. Insert the cloves into the holes leaving the wider part resting on the orange's skin.

5. Tie the ribbon around the orange, like you would a present, you can either tie this in a bow and add some more ribbon or string to hang it from or leave a length for this purpose. (some people prefer to add the ribbon at the start and work around it.)

Be sure to think about your intention whilst making it to add extra power to the pomander.

They also make nice Christmas decorations and gifts.

Definitions

Type	Action
Abortifacient	Can cause an abortion or miscarriage.
Analgesic	Relieves or soothes pain.
Aphrodisiac	Increases sex drive.
Anaesthetic	Reduces or deadens physical sensations.
Antacid	Corrects acidity.
Anti-arthritic	Relieves the symptoms of arthritis
Anti-asthmatic	Relieves the symptoms of asthma.
Antibacterial	Fights bacteria.
Antibiotic	Inhibits the growth of germs, bacteria, and harmful microbes.
Antidepressant	Prevents or wards off depression.
Anti-diarrhoea	Cures diarrhoea.
Antidote	Counteracts poison.
Antifungal	Inhibits and kills various fungi.
Antihistamine	Relieves allergies and hay fever
Anti-inflammatory	Reduce inflammation.
Anti-nausea	Relieves sickness and vomiting
Antioxidant	Wards off negative results of oxidation on body tissues.
Antipyretic	Reduces fever by drawing out the heat.
Anti-rheumatic	Relieves rheumatism.
Antiseptic	Inhibits the growth of micro-organisms.
Antispasmodic	Prevents or relieves muscle spasms
Antitussive	Relieves coughing
Antiviral	Fights viruses.
Astringent	Causes contraction of blood vessels, and tissues where applied, thus can reduce bleeding.
Bitter	Reduces toxins and inflammation. Fights infection, fever, and inflammation
Bitter-tonic	Increases appetite and promotes digestion. Can assist in toning digestive muscles.
Bronchodilator	Opens the bronchi (the upper part

	of the lungs) improving breathing
Carminative	Produces a calming effect on the mind and nerves. Reduces tension and anxiety.
Cardiac	Benefits the heart
Cathartic	Softening stools and helps bowel movement
Cholagogue	Increases the flow of bile.
Decongestant	Relieves nasal congestion
Demulcent	Relieves or soothes pain of inflammation especially in the bladder, gut, sinuses, and stomach.
Depurative	Purifies and cleanses the blood.
Diaphoretic	Promotes perspiration and circulation.
Digestive	Assists with digestion.
Disinfectant	Inhibits or kills disease-producing micro-organisms.
Diuretic	Increases the flow of urine
Emetic	Induce vomiting.
Emmenagogue	Encourages menstrual flow.
Emollient	Soften and soothes irritated skin, inflamed tissue, and mucous membranes.
Expectorant	Expels mucus from the lungs, nose, and throat.
Galactagogue	Helps to increase milk production
Immunostimulant	Helps boost the body's natural immune defences
Laxative	Encourages bowel movement
Purgative	Used to relieve severe constipation
Refrigerant	Relieves fever and thirst. Has cooling properties which help lowers body temperature.
Relaxant	Helps relax and relieve tension, particular effective on muscles.
Rubefacient	Stimulate and increase the blood flow to the surface. Can cause redness to the skin.
Sedative	Possesses calming relaxing effects.
Soporific	Helps promote sleep.
Stimulant	Herb that increases activity. Could be physical mental or organ

	specific.
Tonic	Restores and strengthens the entire system. Promotes well-being
Vasoconstrictor	Constricts the blood vessels and raises blood pressure.
Vasodilator	Expands blood vessels and lowers blood pressure.
Vulnerary	Promotes healing when applied as poultice to fresh cuts and wounds.

Resources

Books:

Bartram's Encyclopaedia of Herbal Medicine - by Thomas Bartram

Holistic herbal: a safe and practical guide to making and using herbal remedies - David Hoffmann

The Book of Herbal Wisdom: Using Plants as Medicine - Matthew Wood

The Apothecary's Garden: How to Grow and Use Your Own Herbal Medicines - Anne McIntyre

The Herbal Home Remedy Book - Joyce A Wardwell

Discover Herbal Remedies: Natural Remedies at Home - Darryl M Smith

Grow Your Own Drugs - James Wong

Natural Healing with Herbs - Humbart Santillo

Healing wise - Susun S Weed

Websites:

http://herbalriot.tumblr.com

http://missionscience.nasa.gov/ems/12_gammarays.html

http://naturalmagickshop.com

http://static.howstuffworks.com

http://store.newwayherbs.com

http://store.newwayherbs.com/

http://toadhollowbeads.com

http://www.bpsmedicine.com/content/7/1/12/abstract

http://www.bristolbotanicals.co.uk

http://www.delhiseeds.org

http://www.flowerempowerment.com

http://www.grannygood.com/

http://www.greathomeremedies.com

http://www.happynaturaltherapies.com

http://www.herbies-herbs.com

http://www.hindawi.com/journals/ecam/2013/361832/

http://www.hindawi.com/journals/ecam/2015/316706/

http://www.jctexports.com

http://www.keeperofthehome.org

http://www.livestrong.com/article/291516-what-are-the-benefits-of-spanish-moss/

http://www.oller.net/incense-making-1.htm

http://www.shirleys-wellness-cafe.com

http://www.somaluna.com

http://www.susunweed.com

http://www.swsbm.com

http://www.thehedgewitchcooks.co.uk

http://www.thevillagewitch.co.uk/

http://www.touchofnatureny.com

https://www.mountainroseherbs.com

https://www.organicfacts.net

Relevant Study Courses:

Aromatherapy

Colour therapy

Herbal Practitioner

Herbal medicine

Holistic therapy diploma

Indian head massage.

Massage therapy

Dear reader,

We hope you enjoyed reading *Herbal Lore*. Please take a moment to leave a review in Amazon, even if it's a short one. Your opinion is important to us.

Discover more books by K.J. Simmill at https://www.nextchapter.pub/authors/kj-simmill

Want to know when one of our books is free or discounted for Kindle? Join the newsletter at http://eepurl.com/bqqB3H

Best regards,

K.J. Simmill and the Next Chapter Team

About the Author

K.J. Simmill is a British author with books released in both the fantasy and non-fiction genres.

She is a qualified Project Manager and Usui Reiki master, with certifications in various fields of holistic therapy. inclusive of aromatherapy, crystal healing, colour therapy, ethereal Reiki, Indian head massage, shaman power Reiki, sound therapy, and massage therapy. She has spent many years researching various practises of magic and herbal medicine and is a qualified herbal practitioner.

When she is not writing, she is an avid reader and a passionate gamer.

You might also like
The Severaine by K.J. Simmill

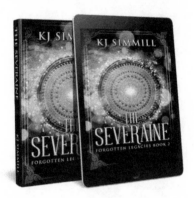

Click here to read the first chapter for free

Herbal Lore
ISBN: 978-4-86747-695-6

Published by
Next Chapter
1-60-20 Minami-Otsuka
170-0005 Toshima-Ku, Tokyo
+818035793528

24th May 2021